take up
PATCHWORK

IONNE HAMMOND

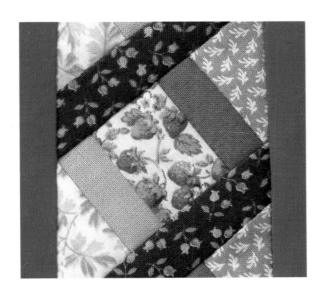

KÖNEMANN

I would like to dedicate this book to
my children, Justin and Erica, for their
support and encouragement in recent
times, and also to David and Dale in
Cincinnati for giving me the courage
to find myself.

Published in 1994 by
Merehurst Limited
Ferry House, 51 – 57 Lacy Road
Putney, London SW 15 1PR

Edited by Alison Wormleighton
Designed by Kit Johnson
Photography by Di Lewis
Illustrations by Paul Bryant

Typesetting by
Litho Link Limited, Welshpool, Powys
Colour seperation by
Fotographics Limited,
UK – Hong Kong

Copyright © 1999 for this edition
Könemann Verlagsgesellschaft mbH
Bonner Str. 126, D- 50968 Cologne

Production Manager: Detlev Schaper
Assistants: Nicola Leurs, Alexandra Kiesling
Printing and Binding:
Sing Cheong Printing Co Ltd., Hong Kong
Printed in Hong Kong China

ISBN 3-8290-2783-4
10 9 8 7 6 5 4 3 2 1

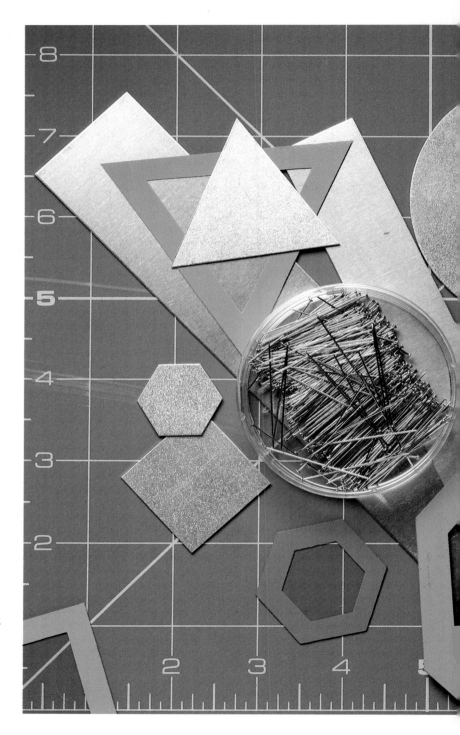

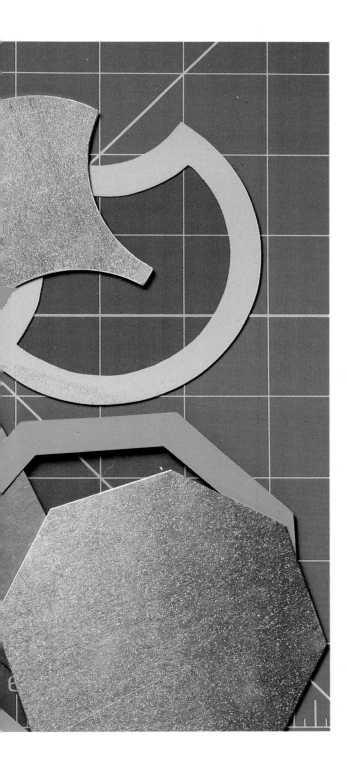

CONTENTS

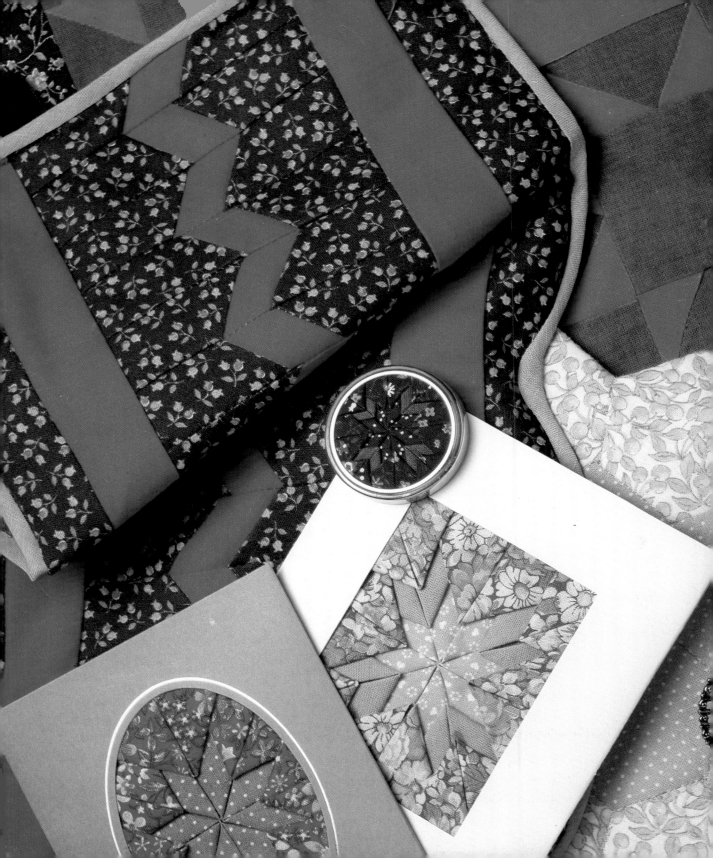

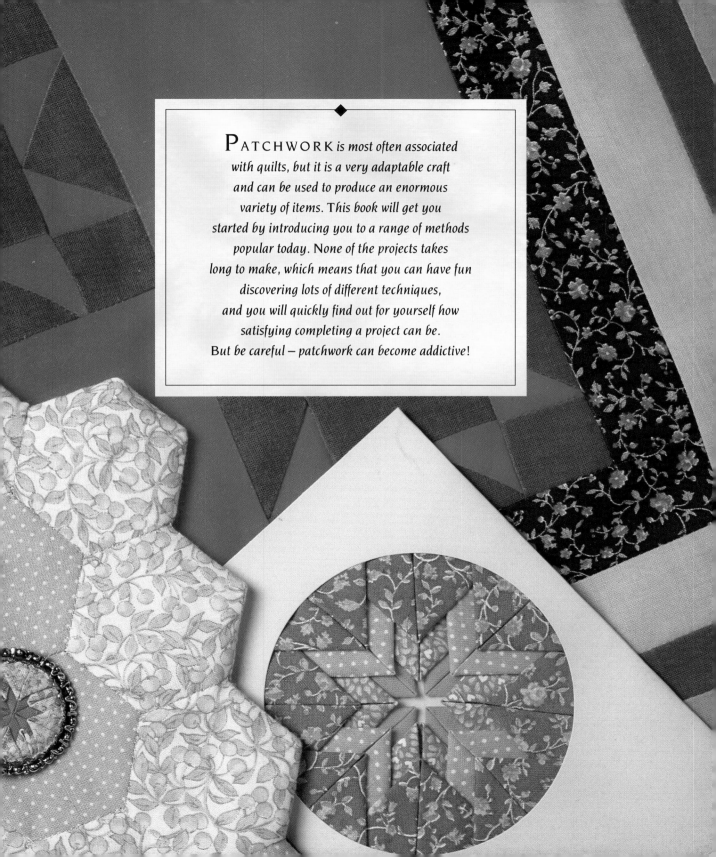

PATCHWORK is most often associated
with quilts, but it is a very adaptable craft
and can be used to produce an enormous
variety of items. This book will get you
started by introducing you to a range of methods
popular today. None of the projects takes
long to make, which means that you can have fun
discovering lots of different techniques,
and you will quickly find out for yourself how
satisfying completing a project can be.
But be careful – patchwork can become addictive!

INTRODUCTION

*The true origins of patchwork are not known but there is
no doubt that through the ages it has developed into an intricate
folk art which continues to fascinate needleworkers of
each successive generation.*

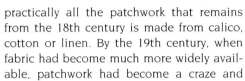

Patchwork has enjoyed enormous popularity for the past two centuries or so, but its history goes back much further. Nowadays, patchwork is more often done for pleasure, as a rewarding creative outlet, and from predominantly new fabrics. But it originally grew out of the need for economy when fabric was a luxury and every remnant was put to good use.

Early patchwork

The earliest known piece of patchwork, an Egyptian ceremonial canopy made of dyed gazelle hide cut into many different patterns, dates from 980 BC. In India pieces of patchwork, believed to be over 1000 years old, have been found; made from many coloured rectangles of silk, they were constructed in exactly the same way as today.

Patchwork began as a thrifty way of reusing the less worn parts of old clothing and furnishing fabrics, and the earliest patchwork quilts were probably made from wool. However, in England in the 17th century, hand-painted, hand-printed cottons began to be imported from India. Brightly coloured and colourfast when washed, they instantly became popular. To protect the weaving trade, embargoes were placed on their import, which led to higher prices. Too valuable to throw away, scraps of this cotton were used to make patchwork furnishings.

A quilt known as the Levens Hall Quilt is the only quilt now in existence made from these imported Indian cottons. Dating from 1708, it is the earliest surviving example of English patchwork. In fact,

practically all the patchwork that remains from the 18th century is made from calico, cotton or linen. By the 19th century, when fabric had become much more widely available, patchwork had become a craze and quilts and coverlets were made by rich and poor alike. Medallion quilts, which had a striking central design, became particularly fashionable. By this time, patchwork was also being used for other purposes, especially chair seat, footstool and cushion covers, tablecloths, bags and antimacassars (covers for the backs and arms of chairs). Previously rare, silks and velvets began to be widely used in patchwork.

American traditions

The American patchwork tradition began with 18th century immigrants from England and continental Europe, who brought the patchwork techniques – and fabrics – with them to the New World. Gradually adapting their needlework to suit the pioneer lifestyle, they used traditional designs but also developed a wealth of new ones.

Many of these designs, such as Wagon Tracks, Cactus Flower and Moon over the Mountain, reflected their lives and the landscape they discovered as they moved west. Other American patterns – with names like Kansas Trouble, Indian Hatchet, Lincoln's Platform and Courthouse Steps – were inspired by everyday objects and forms, as well as social, political, historical and biblical events.

In contrast to English patchwork, which has relatively few traditional names, American patchwork patterns are always given names. These vary according to the locality in which they are made, so that some designs have a number of different ones. Many of the block designs, with intriguing names like Seesaw, Ohio Star and Step to the Altar, drew their inspiration from the ancient craft of paper-folding.

Patchwork quilts

By the end of the 19th century, quilting bees, where the completed patchwork was quilted, were important social events in America. 'Album' quilts, in which each block was worked by a different person, were often assembled on these occasions to be given as gifts. Quilts were a way of expressing friendship or celebrating an event such as a marriage, and their completion was usually accompanied by a party.

Probably the best-known examples of American patchwork are the quilts made by the Amish, with their strikingly simple, abstract designs and stunning colour combinations. These very modern-looking designs are all the more surprising because the Amish are a strict, fundamentalist sect whose members shun the outside world and live very simple lives. Their homes are furnished plainly, with the only source of colour their brightly hued quilts of solid colour (prints being rejected as too worldly). Amish quilts are still being made today, though few are in distinctively Amish designs.

Renewed popularity

Sadly, patchwork went out of favour everywhere at the beginning of the 20th century. It was considered old-fashioned, and many old quilts were discarded or cut up. Today, however, it is enjoying renewed popularity. There is great enjoyment in rediscovering old patterns as well as inventing new ones, and it has become an art form in its own right.

Using this book

This book covers lots of different types of patchwork, so decide which interests you most initially; there is no need to start at the beginning, although you should read pages 10–13 before commencing.

For each type of patchwork, you will find one or two projects. The first is an easy starter project, and when there is a second it uses the same method but is a little more difficult. The final project in the book is made from silk and is best done after you have built up a bit of experience by trying some of the other projects.

On page 68 you will find a Glossary, which explains how to do basic stitches used in patchwork, such as oversewing and running stitch.

Don't be afraid to experiment with your own colour schemes. This has a great deal to do with the fascination of patchwork, as it makes each piece totally individual – a reflection of you. Have fun!

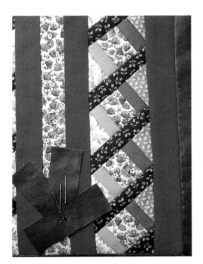
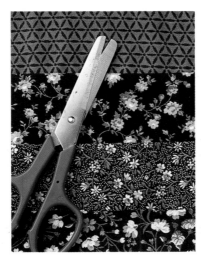
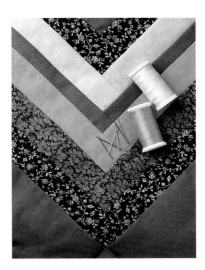

EQUIPMENT AND MATERIALS

*You will probably have many of the articles you need
already in your sewing kit or around the house, but there are
some pieces of specialist equipment which, although not essential,
can make everything much easier.*

Scissors

You will need an extremely sharp pair of dressmaker's shears for cutting your fabric, and if you are using papers you will also need a second pair of scissors to cut them out. Do not even be tempted to use the same pair for both tasks, as the paper would very quickly blunt the blades.

Pins and needles

Long, fine pins such as those used for wedding dresses or lacemaking are best.

When sewing by hand, your stitches usually need to be as small as possible, so you will need to use a fine needle (about size 9 or 10). For machine sewing, use a medium needle (size 14).

Thread

For sewing patches together by hand, use a cotton thread; No. 50 or 60 is ideal. Some patchwork, such as Suffolk Puffs (see page 40), requires a much stronger thread – an extra-strong cotton quilting thread is ideal for this. For machine stitching use a No. 40 cotton thread or a cotton-covered polyester. The thread can match the fabric, or match the darkest fabric, or be in a neutral colour.

Fabric

Always use good-quality fabric. Materials that do not stretch or fray are the easiest to use, and cotton is the

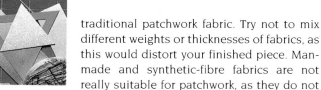

traditional patchwork fabric. Try not to mix different weights or thicknesses of fabrics, as this would distort your finished piece. Man-made and synthetic-fibre fabrics are not really suitable for patchwork, as they do not crease well and are difficult to fold or match accurately. Silk should always be used on its own. Bear in mind that although it looks wonderful, it will not have the lasting quality of cotton.

You may have a particular colour scheme in mind and wish to buy new fabrics, but this will not always be the case. Become a hoarder! Keep scraps of fabric left over from dressmaking, beg from friends and relatives and watch for remnants in sales. You may even want to keep scraps of special fabrics that have a personal or sentimental significance – for example, from old clothes – which can then be sewn into a new article. Your scrap bag can be an inspiration! Avoid mixing old and new fabrics, however, as the stronger fabric will wear out the weaker one.

Templates

These are the reusable patterns used for cutting out patches. You can make your own from cardboard, particularly for simple shapes, but they must be accurate. Metal or plastic templates are available in a wide variety of shapes and sizes in craft shops and from patchwork suppliers. Templates for complex designs that require several shapes are sold as sets.

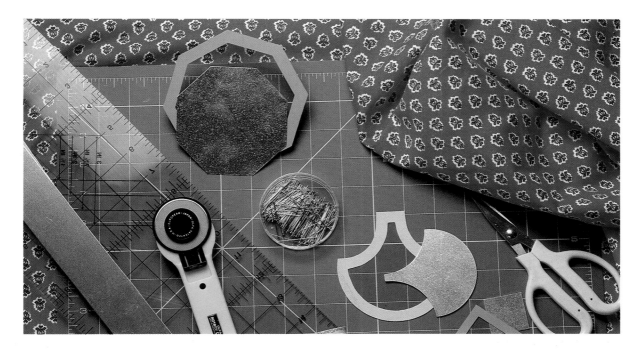

Templates are usually sold in pairs. The smaller, solid shape, which is the size of the finished patch, is used to mark seamlines on patches or to cut papers, depending on the method you are using. The window template, which is the size of the finished patch plus a seam allowance all around, is used for cutting the fabric. The window template is clear in the centre so that it is easy to position on the fabric; you may wish, for example, to centralize a motif such as a single flower. Some templates come with the centre cut out; you draw around the outer edge of these for the fabric shapes and around the inner edge for the seamlines or the papers.

Markers

The marker you use to draw around templates onto fabric must be sharp. You can use an ordinary pencil, pale blue, yellow or white pencils or a dressmaker's pencil. Most pencil marks will wash out. Water-soluble pens are sometimes used, but this ink does not always wash out completely. A fade-away pen, containing disappearing ink, is handy; the lines just fade away after 24 hours.

Specialist accessories

If you are going to make your own templates, you will need a hard pencil, protractor, compass, metal ruler and craft knife. Strong cardboard or plastic can be used, which is obtainable from specialist suppliers.. You may also like to have graph paper and coloured pencils or felt-tip pens to work out your own designs as you become more proficient.

Two of the most useful extras you can buy if you want to continue with your new hobby are a cutting mat and a rotary cutter. Cutting mats come in varying sizes and are made of a special 'self-healing' material marked with a cutting grid and, sometimes, 45 degree angles. Rotary cutters are sharp enough to cut through several layers of fabric at once, removing the tedium of cutting large numbers of shapes for a big project. Replacement blades are available for these.

Also useful is an accurate specialist ruler made of clear, heavy-duty acrylic which can be used with the rotary cutter. These rulers are available with both metric and Imperial measurements and come in a variety of sizes. They also have bias lines for making 30, 45, 60 and 90 degree cuts.

PATCHWORK BASICS

*In this book you'll find some of the most popular types
of patchwork. The finer points of each technique are covered in the
relevant chapter, but there are certain basics you need
to know before you start.*

Cutting fabric

Even patchwork incorporating simple shapes
like squares and rectangles requires precise
cutting and sewing, so it is advisable always
to use a template when cutting out. If you
are using a template that is the size of the finished
patches, you will need to add a seam allowance; this
is usually 6mm (¼ in). Window templates already
have the seam allowance added.

Lay the washed and ironed fabric on a flat surface
with either the right or the wrong side facing. With a
small print or a plain fabric, the patches can be
placed close together to maximize the use of the
fabric. For a larger design, it may be necessary to be
more careful over the placing of the templates.

As many patches as possible should have the grain
of the fabric running in the same direction – ideally
along the longest edge, to minimize stretching. This
is especially important for large patches. Do not use
selvedges, as they distort the work.

Draw around each shape on the fabric and cut out
with sharp scissors. It is sometimes possible to cut
several layers at once, in which case you need to mark
only the top layer. Accuracy is vital.

Joining patches

There are two basic ways of doing patchwork: with
papers (known as the English method) and without
them (called the American method). The English
method can be used for any shape of patch, including
hexagons (the most popular), and gives precise
edges, corners and points. It involves folding all the

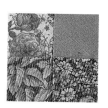

seam allowances of a fabric patch over a
paper shape the size of the finished patch
and basting them in place. The patches are
then sewn together by hand, and the papers
are removed on completion. This method is
explained in detail on pages 34–5. The American
method is suitable for squares, rectangles, triangles
and diamonds and is ideal for block patterns (see
page 16–17). With the American method, the cut-out
patches are placed right sides together and stitched
along the seamline by hand or machine.

Sewing

Patchwork produced without papers can be hand
sewn or machine stitched. Hand sewing makes your
project portable, but machine stitching is quicker and
stronger. You may wish to use both, sewing the
individual patches together into larger units by hand,
then machine stitching these larger units.

If you are using papers, there is no need to mark
seamlines on the patches. But if you are handpiecing
without papers, you will need to mark the seamlines
on the wrong side of the fabric by drawing around a
template that is the finished size of the patches.

Pressing

If you are not using papers, it is important to press
seams as you go, since a seam must always be
pressed before another seam is stitched crossing it.
You can press them open or to one side, but the
latter will make the seams stronger; where possible
press the seam towards the darker fabric.

Order of working

Patchwork is a process of "piecing" – sewing patches together into bigger units, then joining those units into larger units still, and so on. The type of patchwork and the pattern determine the order of piecing.

One of the simplest forms of patchwork involves joining patches into an all-over pattern, creating a mosaic effect. Often it uses only one shape, such as a square or rectangle; the patches are simply joined into strips which are then stitched together.

JOINING PATCHES BY THE AMERICAN METHOD

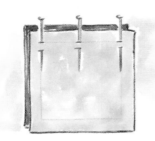

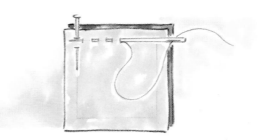

1 ◆ When using the American method of patchwork (ie with no papers), pin the fabric patches together with right sides facing and the edges even. Place pins on the seamline and at points where seamlines meet, as shown. For long patches, you will probably also need one or more pins in between.

2 ◆ For hand sewing, use a small running stitch – about 3–4 stitches to the centimetre (8–10 stitches to the inch). Start and finish with a few backstitches. For machine stitching use a medium-length stitch – about 5 stitches to the centimetre (12 stitches to the inch). Remove the pins as you approach.

PIECING A MOSAIC DESIGN

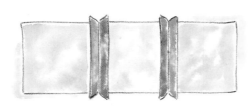

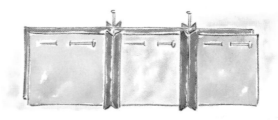

1 ◆ To join patches to form a mosaic design, sew the first two patches together, taking a 6mm (¼in) seam allowance. Press the seam open or to one side. Join another patch to the first two, then another and so on, until the strip is the width of the design. Join the remaining patches into strips in the same way.

2 ◆ To complete the design, pin one strip to another with right sides facing, taking great care to match the seams at right angles to the edge you are sewing. Stitch the two strips together. Attach another strip in the same way, and continue until all the strips are joined. Press the seams open or to the side.

SQUARE DEAL

*Patchwork makes brilliant curtains! And the technique
of joining squares to form an all-over pattern is so quick and
easy that even quite large curtains are possible.*

SIZE

Each of the 2 curtains
measures 93cm (36½ in)
square. You could alter the
size by using a different
number of patches or
patches of a different size.

YOU WILL NEED

2m (2⅛ yd) of peach chintz
122cm (48in) wide

25cm (¼ yd) each of 2 plain
fabrics in green and pink

25cm (¼ yd) each of 10
patterned fabrics in greens,
peaches and pinks

2m (2⅛ yd) of curtain
heading tape

Matching thread

4 brass curtain rings

Small amount of wadding
(batting) for stuffing tie-
backs

PREPARATION

1 ◆ Using the square template on
page 60, cut 81 fabric squares for
each curtain. The template
includes a 6mm (¼ in) seam
allowance all around.

2 ◆ Lay the fabric patches out in a
square 9 patches across by 9
patches down. Move the patches
around until you achieve your
required design, trying not to
repeat any fabric in the lines
across or down – this is not as
easy as it looks! Keep checking
until you are sure. Reverse the
design for the second curtain.

JOINING THE PATCHES

1 ◆ With right sides together, join
each of the 9 patches in the first
row to its neighbour, taking a
6mm (¼ in) seam. Repeat for the
other 8 rows. You should now
have 9 strips.

2 ◆ Join the strips to each other,
taking great care to pin and baste
first so that the seams match
accurately.

3 ◆ Repeat the process for the
other curtain.

MAKING UP

1 ◆ Cut 2 pieces of chintz the
same size as each curtain.

2 ◆ Place a curtain and a piece of
chintz right sides together, and
stitch a 6mm (¼ in) seam along
one side, along the bottom and
up the other side, leaving the top
edges unstitched.

3 ◆ Trim 2.5cm (1in) from the
chintz at the top. Turn under 6mm
(¼ in) at the top of the patchwork
and attach the curtain heading
tape, machine stitching along
both edges of the tape and across
the ends.

4 ◆ Complete the other curtain in
the same way.

CURTAIN TIE-BACKS

1 ◆ Cut 2 strips each of peach
chintz, plain fabric and print
fabric, all 48cm (19in) × 4.5cm
(1¾ in), and 4 strips of peach
chintz 6cm (2⅜ in) × 8.5cm
(3⅜ in).

2 ◆ Fold each of the 6 long strips
in half lengthwise, right sides
together. Sew across one end and
down the long side, taking a 6mm
(¼ in) seam. Turn right side out
and stuff with wadding (batting).
Stitch the open end closed.

3 ◆ Sew 3 stuffed strips, 1 in each
fabric, together at one end. Plait
(braid) the strips and then sew
them together at the other end.
Repeat for the other 3 strips.

4 ◆ To make endpieces for the tie-
backs, fold each of the short strips
in half crosswise, right sides
together. Stitch a 1cm (⅜ in)
seam down each side of the

folded strip; the seam is wider than usual to make it stronger. Turn right side out.

5 ◆ Slot each endpiece over one end of the tie-backs. Turn under 6mm (¼ in) all around the raw edge of each and slip-stitch in place by hand.

6 ◆ Sew a curtain ring to each end of the tie-backs.

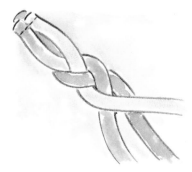

◆ *Plaiting (braiding) three stuffed strips to make one tie-back*

◆ *Endpiece for tie-back*

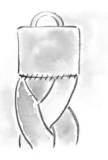

◆ *Endpiece slotted over plait and slip-stitched in place; curtain ring sewn on*

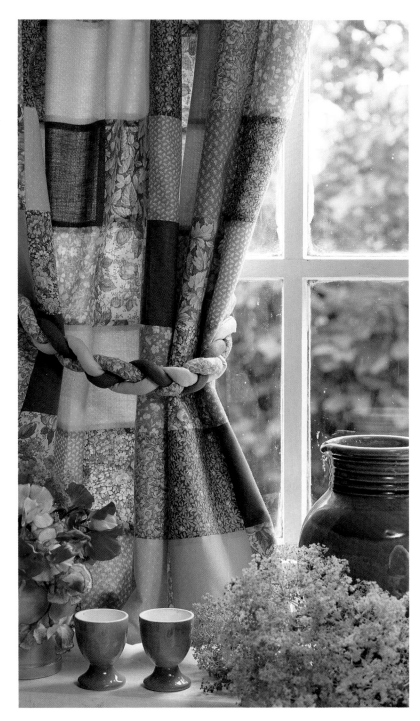

BLOCKS AND MEDALLIONS

*With this type of patchwork an infinite variety of designs
can be built up from geometric shapes. Even quite large pieces
can be made relatively quickly by someone with
little sewing experience.*

Pieced blocks

This technique, which is much used in the United States, involves piecing patches together into 'blocks' usually square in shape, which are then sewn together (called 'setting'). Although blocks vary in size considerably, the average block is about 25–30cm (10–12in) square.

The blocks may be joined edge-to-edge to form one unbroken design, or they may be separated by strips of fabric (variously known as sashes, lattice bands, linking strips or dividers). Turning the blocks 45 degrees (called 'setting them on point') is also common. Blocks may be all the same design or different; sometimes design blocks are alternated with plain ones.

Most block designs belong to either the four-patch or the nine-patch family. They consist of four or nine basic units, which may be subdivided in various ways, for example into triangles. There is no maximum number of patches in the block, but the total is always divisible by four or nine respectively.

Other block patterns include five-patch and seven-patch designs; with these, however, the names refer to the number of units across and down. In other words, a five-patch block consists of 25 units – five across and five down.

There is a huge variety of designs which have been handed down through the ages, with evocative names like Sunshine and Shadow, Old Maid's Puzzle, Bear's

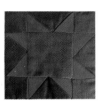

Paw, Farmer's Daughter, Monkey Wrench and Streak O'Lightning. Straight lines and geometric shapes characterize this type of patchwork, and it is therefore ideally suited to the American method of joining patches (see pages 12–13). The English method, using papers (see page 34), is also suitable for block patchwork, but it is usually only employed for very small patches since the American method is so much faster and just as effective for this type of patchwork.

Patches are joined in basically the same way as for mosaic designs (see page 13). Triangles are first joined to form squares, then the squares are joined into rows, and the rows into blocks. The blocks are then sewn together, or sewn to sashes, depending on the particular design.

Medallion designs

Some designs consist of blocks which together form a central motif and are surrounded by borders that 'frame' the motif. These are known as medallion designs. The centrepiece isn't necessarily made from pieced blocks – it may instead consist of one piece of fabric or perhaps a quilted or appliquéd motif.

Medallion quilts were popular early in the 19th century, when it was fashionable for the central panels to commemorate historic events. Specially printed panels were available for this. Embroidery was also sometimes used for the central motif.

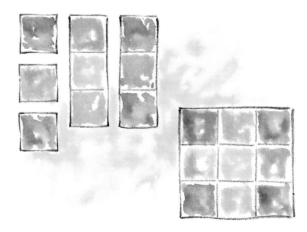

1 ◆ Plan the order of piecing for a block so that all the seams are straight and so that you can avoid having to stitch L-shaped seams.

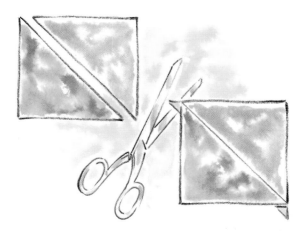

2 ◆ Start by joining the smallest patches – for example, stitching two triangles to form a square. After pressing the seam to one side, snip off the 'tails' (protruding seam allowances).

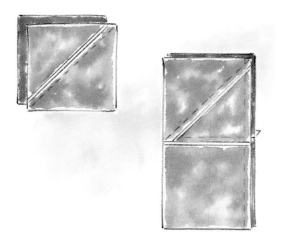

3 ◆ Stitch these pieces together into larger units – for example, joining two squares to form a rectangle. Continue joining larger and larger units until the block is complete.

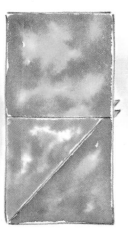

4 ◆ Note that when you stitch a square consisting of two triangles to another square, the point of the triangle on the seamline will be 6mm (¼ in) away from the raw edge that is at right angles to it. Then, when that raw edge is also stitched, the point will be exactly on the seamline.

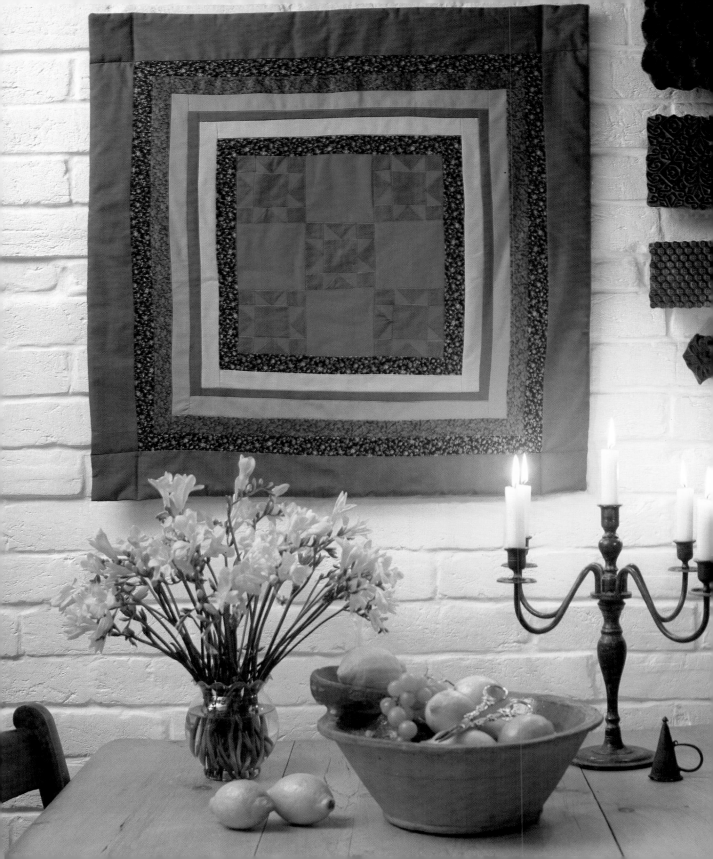

CENTRE OF ATTENTION

*This wall hanging, in a traditional American patchwork
design called Star Medallion, features a centrepiece of four-patch
blocks alternating with plain blocks. The centrepiece
is framed by pieced borders.*

SIZE

The wall hanging measures
84cm (33in) square.

YOU WILL NEED

25cm (¼ yd) each of bright
pink, light green and light
pink fabric 115cm (45in)
wide

50cm (½ yd) of navy/pink
print fabric 115cm (45in)
wide

25cm (¼ yd) of green print
fabric 115cm (45in) wide

1.4m (1½ yd) of dark green
fabric 115cm (45in) wide

Piece of wadding (batting)
1m (1yd) square

Matching threads

6 curtain rings

82.5cm (32½ in) dowel

String

PREPARATION

Using the templates on page 61,
cut the following pieces. These
dimensions include a 6mm (¼in)
seam allowance all around.

Medium squares: cut 5 from dark
green

Small squares: cut 20 from dark
green

Large triangles: cut 20 from dark
green

Small triangles: cut 40 from
bright pink

Large squares: cut 4 from bright
pink

Measure and cut the following
border strips:

5cm (2in) × 31.8cm (12½ in)
border strips A: cut 2 from navy/
pink print

5cm (2 in) × 39.4cm (15½ in)
border strips A: cut 2 from navy/
pink print

5cm (2in) × 39.4cm (15½ in)
border strips B: cut 2 from light
green

5cm (2in) × 47cm (18½ in) border
strips B: cut 2 from light green

3.8 cm (1½ in) × 47cm (18½ in)
border strips C: cut 2 from dark
green

3.8 cm (1½ in) × 52cm (20½ in)
border strips C: cut 2 from dark
green

5cm (2in) × 52cm (20½ in)
border strips D: cut 2 from light
pink

5cm (2in) × 59.7cm (23½ in)
border strips D: cut 2 from light
pink

5cm (2in) × 59.7cm (23½ in)
border strips E: cut 2 from green
print

5cm (2in) × 67.3cm (26½ in)
border strips E: cut 2 from green
print

5cm (2in) × 57.3cm (26½ in)
border strips F: cut 2 from navy/
pink print

5cm (2in) × 74.9cm (29½ in)
border strips F: cut 2 from navy/
pink print

8.2cm (3¼ in) × 74.9cm (29½ in)
border strips G: cut 2 from dark
green

8.2cm (3¼ in) × 81.9cm (32¼in)
border strips G: cut 2 from dark
green

JOINING THE PATCHES

There are 5 design blocks, each
pieced as follows.

1 ◆ Sew one green triangle to 2
pink ones, forming a rectangle.

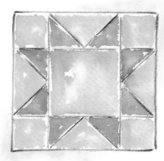

◆ *One pieced block*

2 ◆ Make 3 more rectangles. Join one of these rectangles to the top of a medium dark green square and another rectangle to the bottom, points outwards.
3 ◆ Join a small dark green square to each end of a third rectangle. Repeat for 2 more dark green squares and the fourth rectangle.
4 ◆ Now join the 3 pieces to form one block. Repeat steps 2–4 for 4 more blocks.
5 ◆ Create a chequerboard pattern for the central motif as follows. Sew 2 design blocks to a bright pink square to make a strip. Make another strip in the same way. Make a third strip by sewing the remaining design block to the 2 remaining bright pink squares. Stitch the first two strips on either side of this strip.
6 ◆ Add the 7 sets of borders; work from the centre outwards, starting with border strips A and finishing with G. For each set, stitch the 2 shorter ones on either end first, then the two longer ones on either side. Press very carefully.

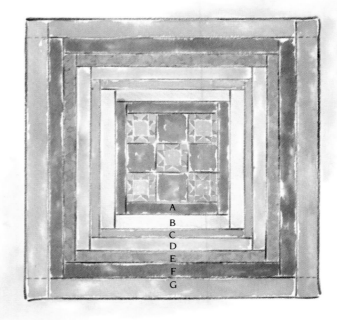

◆ *Central motif made up of five pieced blocks and four plain ones in chequerboard pattern, surrounded by series of border strips*

MAKING UP
1 ◆ Cut a piece of wadding (batting) which is the same size as the completed patchwork. Place it on the wrong side and baste through both thicknesses with large stitches.
2 ◆ Cut a piece of dark green fabric the same size as the completed patchwork. With right sides together, join the fabric to the patchwork by stitching a 6mm (¼ in) seam all around, leaving a 10cm (4in) opening at the centre of one side.
3 ◆ Turn the hanging right side out through the opening. Neatly slip-

stitch the opening closed, and press the edges.
4 ◆ The hanging can be quilted as much or as little as you wish; our hanging has a simple square stitched at each corner. Baste around the edges and in about 5 parallel rows across the hanging, then stitch through all layers along the seamlines.
5 ◆ Sew 6 curtain rings to the back of the hanging at the top edge, spacing them evenly. Slot the length of dowelling through the rings, and tie a piece of string to the dowelling for hanging.

◆ *The Star Medallion wall hanging is padded, but if you do not wish to hang your work, it could be made without the padding and used as a table centrepiece (opposite).*

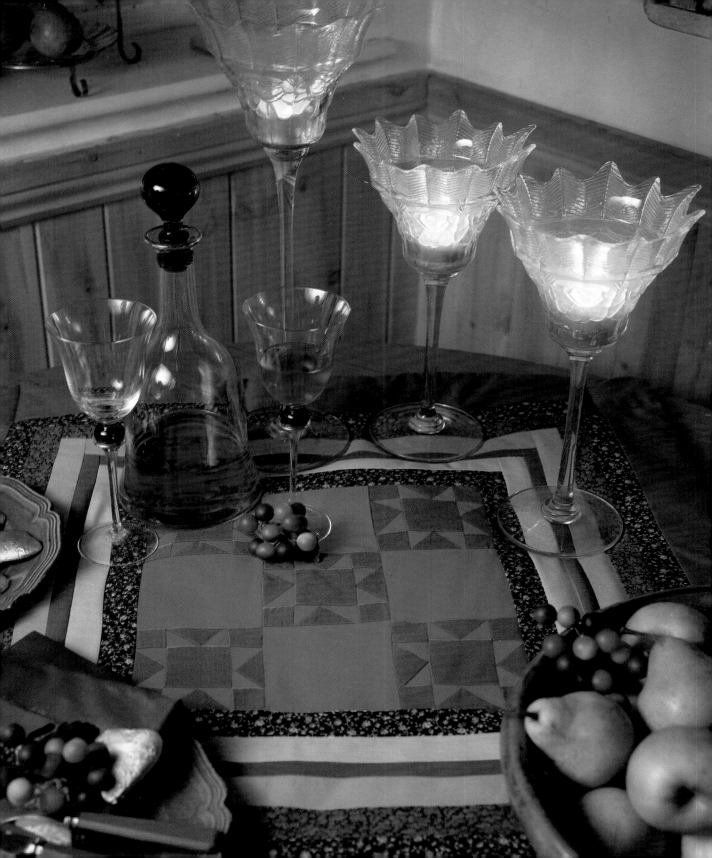

SEMINOLE PATCHWORK

*For nearly a century, the Seminole Indians of
Florida have decorated their clothing with bands of vividly
coloured patchwork, and the same method can be used for a
variety of purposes in the home as well.*

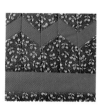

Seminole patchwork can be made using plain or patterned fabrics, or a combination of both, but it is most striking with plain fabrics in bold colours. This is because the technique of sewing, cutting and rejoining several times emphasizes the colours and produces dramatic contrasts. The patches may look quite tiny, yet they are actually easy to handle because they are always in strips.

This is a fundamentally modern form of patchwork and, although it is possible to sew it by hand, it is best made on the machine – for which it was actually developed – and will produce a very quick, attractive and unusual result.

Choosing fabrics

You will need to carry out a few experiments before you reach a final design, as it is difficult to see the effect you will produce with your chosen fabrics unless you sew a few sample pieces first. Try several different combinations of fabric and compare the results before making a decision. Even just three fabrics will produce a huge number of different designs, but you can, of course, use as many fabrics as you wish.

The choice of colour and the arrangement of fabric are both important factors and it is worth spending some time experimenting with different colours and layouts before starting. The more you use of one particular colour, the stronger it will appear in your finished article. Remember that dominant colours like reds and yellows will stand out more than blues and greens, so if you want to emphasize a particular part of a blue and yellow design, for example, use the yellow where you want the emphasis to be. Another factor to keep in mind is that there are many seams in Seminole patchwork. Not only will you need more fabric than for most other types of patchwork, but because there are so many seams, it is important to use a lightweight fabric such as cotton lawn that will press easily and not fray. Wonderful colours and textures can be obtained using silk but you need more experience for this, as fraying can be a problem.

Cutting and joining the strips

With this technique in particular it is important to cut the fabric strips on the grain, from selvedge to selvedge, otherwise the fabric will stretch unevenly and accurate joining will be impossible. Seams are pressed to one side rather than open, and must be pressed only gently to avoid stretching.

The width of the strips can vary. If you are using very fine fabrics, they could be as narrow as 2cm (¾in), while for heavier fabrics they could be up to 8cm (3in) or even wider.

All Seminole patterns are created by cutting the joined fabric strips at intervals, either vertically or at angles, then sewing the cut sections together again in new patterns. If desired, bands of fabric can then be joined to the patchwork to link all the patches together. The steps shown opposite are for two particular designs, but the procedure is typical of Seminole patchwork in general.

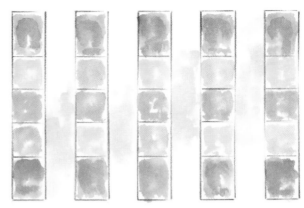

1 ◆ Cutting on the grain of the fabric, cut two strips 4cm (1½ in) wide of colour A. Cut a strip 3cm (1¼ in) wide of colour B, of print C and of print D. Arrange them alongside each other as shown. With right sides facing, stitch adjacent strips together along the long edges, taking 6mm (¼ in) seams. Press the seam allowance gently to one side.

2 ◆ Cut the resulting pieced fabric into 3cm (1¼ in) wide strips, cutting at right angles to the seamlines. Place the new strips side by side, turning each alternate strip the opposite way.

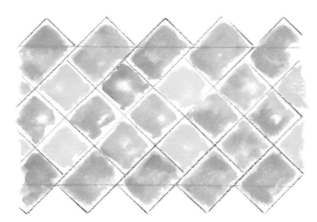

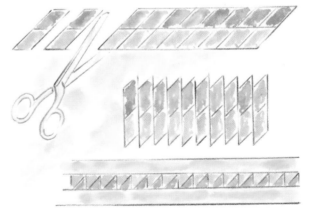

3 ◆ Stagger the strips as shown and sew them together along the long sides, taking 6mm (¼ in) seams. Press the seams to one side. Trim the top and bottom edges 6mm (¼ in) outside the points of colour A to leave a seam allowance.

4 ◆ Here is another design, this time using only two strips. The two strips are joined, cut at an angle of 45 degrees then staggered and rejoined. After the edges are trimmed, a band is added to the top and bottom.

HOT STUFF

Keep your coffee hot with this smart cover for a cafetière
(French press). It's made using Seminole patchwork, a quick and
easy method of creating intricate geometric designs.

SIZE

The cover fits a medium-sized (8-cup) cafetière.

YOU WILL NEED

25cm (¼ yd) each of dark green chintz, dark green/pink print fabric and dark red plain fabric

1.5m (1½ yd) of light green bias binding

5cm (2in) of black touch-and-close fastener

Small piece of wadding (batting)

Matching thread

PREPARATION

Cut the following strips, all 46cm (18in) in length. All the strips should be cut on the straight grain of the fabric. These dimensions include 6mm (¼ in) seam allowances.

4cm (1½ in) wide strips: cut 6 from print fabric and cut 2 from plain red fabric

2cm (¾ in) wide strips: cut 2 from plain red fabric

JOINING THE PATCHES

1 ◆ Make a band by sewing a patterned strip to a narrow plain strip, then sewing another patterned strip to the other side of the plain strip. Make a second band in the same way.

2 ◆ Cut each band into 3cm (1¼ in) sections at an angle of 55 degrees, on opposite diagonals.

3 ◆ Sew the sections together, alternating one section from each band, taking care to match the seams exactly. Trim the top and bottom edges.

4 ◆ Add a wide plain strip and then a patterned strip at the top and bottom of the band.

MAKING UP

1 ◆ Using the pattern on page 58, cut out one cover piece from chintz, one from wadding (batting) and one from the completed patchwork.

2 ◆ Sandwich the 3 layers together with wrong sides facing. Edge with the bias binding.

3 ◆ Cut the touch-and-close fastener into 2 pieces and stitch them at the top and bottom of the cover at appropriate points to allow for the cafetière handle. Press carefully.

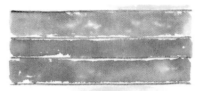

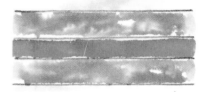

◆ *Sewing 2 bands, each made up of 2 patterned strips and 1 narrow plain strip*

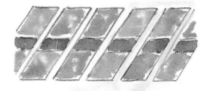

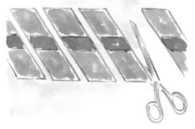

◆ *Cutting each band into 3cm (1¼ in) segments on opposite diagonals*

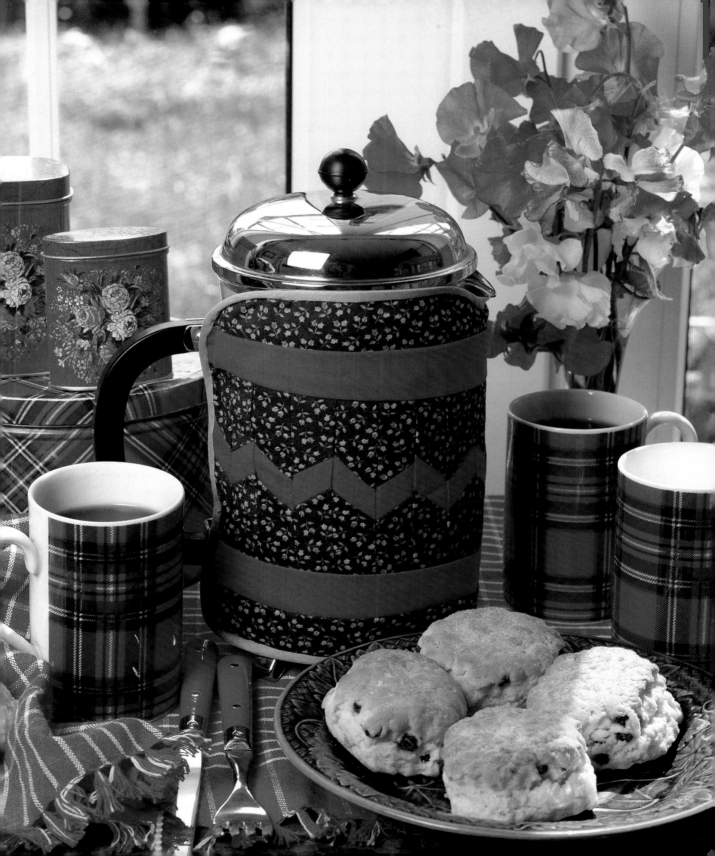

WELL PLACED

The intricate pattern of this placemat looks complicated,
but the Seminole patchwork technique makes it so quick and easy
that you could do a whole set.

SIZE

The placemat measures
43cm (17in) × 30cm (12in).

YOU WILL NEED

50cm (½ yd) of dark green
chintz

25cm (¼ yd) each of light
green, mid green and dark
red plain fabrics, and of 4
different green print fabrics
(prints A, B, C, D)

Piece of wadding (batting)
30cm (12in) × 43cm (17in)

Matching thread

PREPARATION

Cut the following pieces on the
straight grain of the fabric. These
dimensions include 6mm (¼ in)
seam allowances.

3.8cm (1½ in) × 46cm (18in)
strips: cut 2 from each of prints A,
B and C, 4 from the dark red fabric
and 1 from print A, B or C.

2cm (¾ in) × 46cm (18in) strips:
cut 2 each from light green, mid
green and print D.

Cut a 54.6cm (21½ in) × 39.4cm
(15½ in) piece of chintz.

JOINING THE PATCHES

1 ◆ Arrange one of each of the 3
print strips and 2 of the plain
strips as follows: print A, light
green, print B, dark green, print C.
Stitch each strip to the adjacent
ones. This will be used for the
bottom band of the design. Repeat
in reverse for the top band.
2 ◆ Cutting at right angles to the
seamlines, cut each of the 2
patchwork pieces into 14 pieced
strips 3cm (1¼ in) wide.
3 ◆ Cut each of the 2 narrow print
D strips into 14 pieces, each 10cm
(4in) long. With right sides
together, stitch one of these down
the side of each pieced strip.
4 ◆ Stagger the pieced strips for
the top band, and, with right sides
facing, join adjacent strips as
shown in the third diagram.
Repeat for the bottom band.
5 ◆ Trim the top and bottom
edges to leave a 6mm (¼ in)
seam allowance all around the 2
bands. With right sides facing,
stitch a dark red strip to the top
and bottom edges of each band.
6 ◆ With right sides facing, stitch
the top band to one long edge of
the remaining print B strip, and
stitch the bottom band to the
other long edge.

◆ *Sewing strips together to form a band*

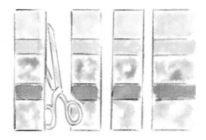

◆ *Cutting a pieced band into strips*

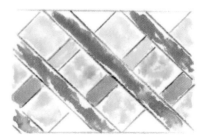

◆ *Sewing a narrow print strip down the side*
of each pieced strip, staggering them and
rejoining, then trimming the edges

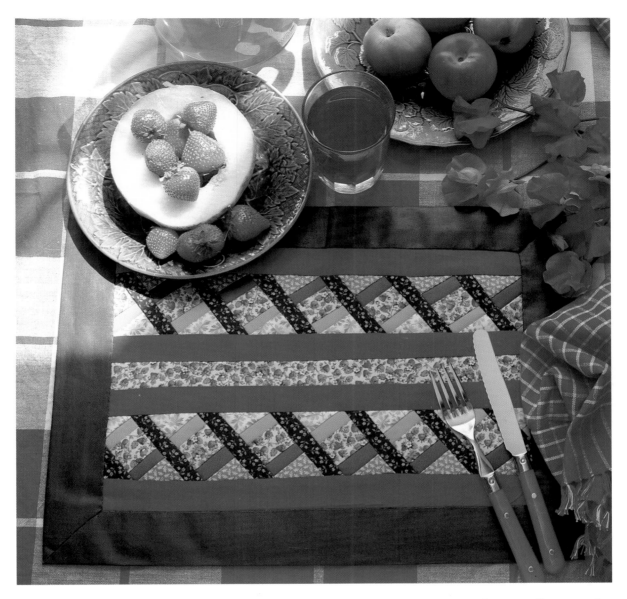

MAKING UP

1 ◆ Trim the edges to form a rectangle 35.5cm (14in) × 23cm (9in). Place it in the centre of the piece of wadding (batting), right side up, and baste through both layers with large stitches.

2 ◆ Place the patchwork and wadding (batting) in the centre of the piece of green chintz, with wrong sides facing. Turn under 6mm (¼ in) along the wrong edges of the chintz.

3 ◆ Fold in all 4 sides of the chintz to cover the seam allowance of the patchwork and create a chintz border all around the mat.

4 ◆ Mitre the corners as shown on page 43, and slip-stitch the chintz to the patchwork. Press the work carefully.

FOLDED STARS

*This type of patchwork creates a three-dimensional effect
that is quite unique, yet it is not at all difficult to do. In England
it is also called Somerset patchwork, and in America
Prairie Points or Mitred patchwork.*

With the Folded Star technique, squares, rectangles or circles of fabric are folded into triangles and attached to a backing fabric to create patterns, particularly star shapes. The backing fabric does not show but it gives strength to the article. This technique offers a great opportunity to experiment with colours and patterns.

You can make your own templates from stiff cardboard or plastic. The triangles can be sewn on by hand or machine, although the points need to be caught down by hand. If the article is to be purely decorative, the triangles can even be glued on with a specialist fabric glue.

It is best to use fine fabrics because the folding and layering of the patches can make it very bulky. It is also helpful if the fabric will crease easily, so pure cotton is best. Ribbon can be used too. The three-dimensional quality of this technique is quite unlike traditional forms of patchwork and adds to its attractiveness. It can be used for many different purposes, from greetings cards to cushions, and even to add decoration to clothing such as jackets or waistcoats.

For the most striking effects, aim for dramatic contrasts. Avoid large-scale patterns – with such small triangles, tiny prints and plain fabrics look best.

Triangles made from rectangles, as shown here, are the most common, but they can also be made from squares and circles, both of which should be folded in half first, rather than turning under 6mm (¼ in). The 'triangles' formed by folded circles actually have curved bases, but the method is the same.

FOLDED STARS FROM RECTANGLES

1 ◆ Mark a square the size of the finished piece on the plain backing fabric. Mark horizontal, vertical and dividing lines. Drawing the lines accurately is important, in order to ensure the correct placing of the fabric triangles.

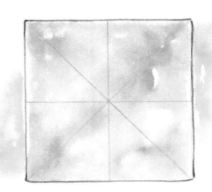

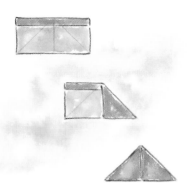

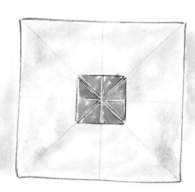

2 ◆ Cut out rectangles from your chosen fabric, all to exactly the same size, cutting on the straight grain. Turn 6mm (¼ in) to the wrong side on the long edge, creasing the fold with your fingernail. Now fold one corner down to the centre, as shown; the bottom edges do not to have to be even. Repeat for the other corner. Make as many triangles as you will need.

3 ◆ For the first round, place the points of four triangles to the centre marked on the backing fabric, folded sides up, using the marked lines as a guide. These points may touch or, if you are using a coloured backing fabric, you may prefer to leave a small gap so that the colour shows through slightly. For each triangle, catch down the centre point with one or two tiny backstitches through all layers. Secure the outer edge with running stitches.

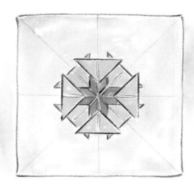

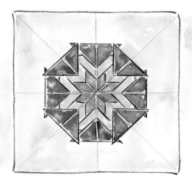

4 ◆ For the second round, lay four more folded triangles over the first four triangles as shown, using the lines marked on the backing fabric, and placing the points an equal distance from the centre. Catch the centre point of each down, and work running stitches along the outer edges as before. Complete the second round by laying four more folded triangles over the other four in that round, as shown. Catch-stitch the centre points and work running stitches around the edges as before

5 ◆ Like the second round, the third round will consist of eight triangles. Any subsequent rounds will require 16 triangles each. Continue adding triangles until you reach the desired size.

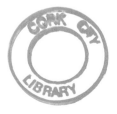

STAR ATTRACTION

*This greetings card will be cherished by the recipient
at least as much as a gift. Choose the fabric to suit the occasion,
from Christmas to a Golden Wedding anniversary.*

SIZE

Card 1 measures 15.2cm (6in) × 10cm (4in) and has an 8.2cm (3¼ in) round aperture.

Card 2 measures 15.2cm (6in) × 10cm (4in) and has a 7.6cm (3in) × 5.7cm (2¼ in) oblong aperture.

Card 3 measures 9cm (3½ in) × 11.5cm (4½ in) and has a 7.6cm (3in) × 5cm (2in) oval aperture.

YOU WILL NEED

Scraps of fabric

Double-fold cards with shaped apertures

Plain fabric (optional)

Matching threads or fabric glue

PREPARATION
Using the template on page 62, cut the following pieces.

For Card 1
5.7cm (2¼ in) × 3.2cm (1¼ in) rectangles: cut 4 each from plain fabric and prints A and B, and 8 from print C.

For Card 2
5.7cm (2¼ in) × 3.2cm (1¼ in) rectangles: cut 4 each from plain fabric and print D, and 8 from print E.

For Card 3
5.7cm (2¼ in) × 3.2cm (1¼ in) rectangles: cut 4 from print F and 8 from print G.

JOINING THE PATCHES
For Card 1
1 ◆ Fold each rectangle into a triangle, as on page 29, step 2.
2 ◆ Mark the centre of the circle and the diagonals on the cardboard backing inside the aperture, and arrange the first 4 triangles of plain fabric as shown on page 29, step 3. Use a little glue to fix the points.
3 ◆ Place the 4 triangles in print A accurately over the gaps between the plain triangles.
4 ◆ Do the same with the 4 triangles in print B, as on page 29, step 4.
5 ◆ Place the first 4 triangles in print C accurately over the print A triangles. Put the remaining 4 print C triangles over the print B ones, slightly overlapping on each side those already placed.

For Card 2
1 ◆ Fold each rectangle into a triangle, as shown on page 29, step 2. Either glue the patches in place or sew them to a backing fabric that is 6mm (¼ in) larger all around than the aperture. If sewing, mark the centre of the backing fabric.
2 ◆ Arrange the triangles with the points meeting at the centre. Catch the points down with 1 or 2 tiny backstitches, and baste along the outer edge of each triangle and the diagonals.
3 ◆ Arrange a second layer of 4 triangles where the first triangles touch.
4 ◆ Follow with the outer layer as for Card 1.

For Card 3
1 ◆ Fold each rectangle into a triangle, as shown on page 29, step 2.
2 ◆ Arrange the first layer as before and follow with a second layer of 8 triangles, finishing in the same way.

MAKING UP
Once the patchwork is complete, close the card behind the aperture and stick it down.

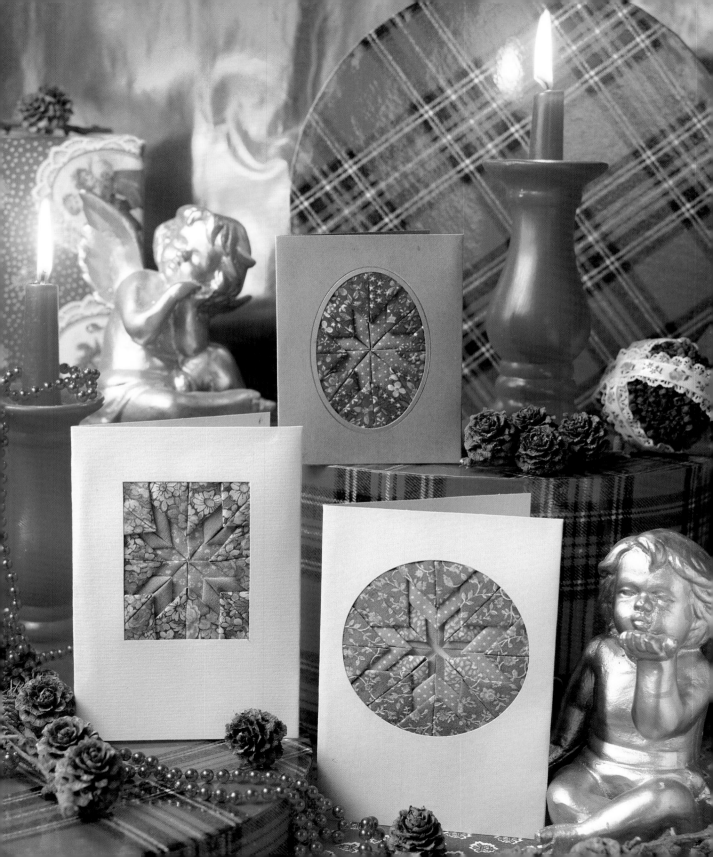

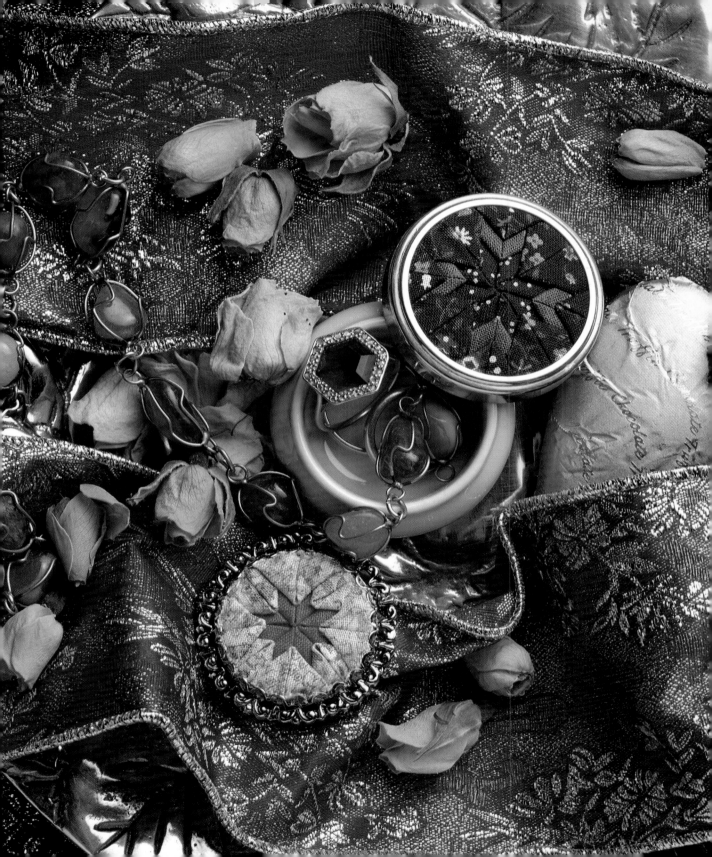

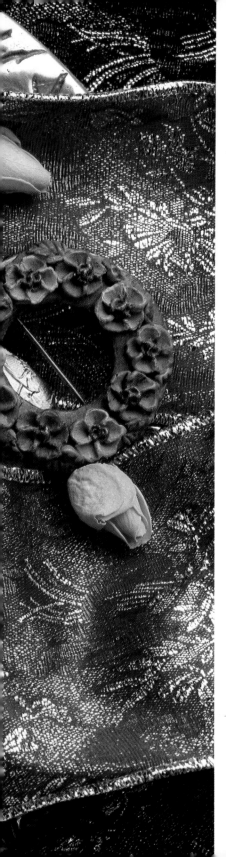

SMALL BUT PERFECT

*Holding the same fascination as miniature
paintings, this tiny trinket box and brooch prove that
small is beautiful too, providing a showcase for your
new skills on a completely different scale than
most other patchwork projects.*

SIZE

The pieced part of the
trinket box lid is 3.2cm
(1¼ in) in diameter. The
pieced area of the brooch is
2.5cm (1in) in diameter.

YOU WILL NEED

Scraps of fabric

China box with 3.8cm
(1½ in) lid

Circular brooch mount

Fabric glue

Clear nail polish (optional)

PREPARATION

Using the template on page 62,
cut the following pieces.

For the trinket box
3.8cm (1½ in) × 2.5cm (1in) rectangles: cut 4 each in plain fabric
and print A, and 8 in print B.

For the brooch
3.8cm (1½ in) × 2.5cm (1in) rectangles: cut 4 in plain fabric and
8 in print fabric.

JOINING THE PATCHES

1 ◆ Use the paper circle which has
been supplied with the box or
brooch as the base for your
design.
2 ◆ Mark the centre of the circle
and arrange the triangles in the
same way as described for Card 2
on page 30.
3 ◆ Glue the point of each triangle
down carefully. The final layer of
triangles will overlap the paper
circle.
4 ◆ When the glue is dry, trim
away excess fabric from around
the edge of the patchwork to
make it the size of the circle, and
press firmly. Place this inside the
metal rim of the box.

MAKING UP

1 ◆ Follow the manufacturer's
instructions for completing the lid
or brooch, but do not use the
acetate circle on the lid as this
would detract from the texture of
the design.
2 ◆ You may find it useful to apply
a touch of clear nail polish
around the edges of the fabric to
prevent fraying.

ENGLISH PATCHWORK

*Using papers inside each shape when joining patches
by hand enables you to create designs using more complicated
shapes. Popular and versatile, this is probably the best-
known type of patchwork in Britain.*

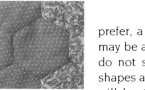

Though less common in Europe and America, this method dates from the early 18th century in England. Because the seam allowances of the patches are folded over papers (and basted together temporarily) and the patches are then oversewn together, shapes such as octagons, pentagons and hexagons can all be used.

Honeycombs and rosettes

The hexagon – a six-sided shape – is the one most associated with English patchwork. When all the sides are the same length, it is also known as a honeycomb.

Hexagons are most often sewn together to form rosettes, which offer innumerable design possibilities. A single rosette is made up of a hexagon surrounded by six others. In a double rosette these are surrounded by 12 more hexagons. The most common pattern, Grandmother's Flower Garden, consists of double rosettes separated by plain hexagons.

Cutting out papers and patches

Although, in the past, newspapers and letters were often used for papers, they really need to be from a stronger paper so they retain their shape and resist the folding of the fabric over them, without being so thick that they are hard to handle or to baste through. Good writing paper or greetings cards are ideal. Using a sharp pencil, draw around the smaller template of the pair (see page 11) onto the paper, angling the pencil into the template to make it exact, then cut out very accurately with paper-cutting scissors (or, if you

prefer, a craft knife and cutting board). You may be able to cut two or three at once, but do not sacrifice accuracy for speed. Fabric shapes are cut using the larger template and will be 6mm (¼ in) larger all around than the papers. Be careful how you cut these to ensure you get the best part of your fabric design in the centre. At least one side of the template should lie on the straight grain of the fabric, and all the patches in one fabric should run in the same direction. There is no need to mark the seamlines.

Sewing the patches together

Each patch is basted to a paper as shown in the steps opposite, and then the edges of the patches are sewn together by hand. Tiny oversewing stitches – 6 to 8 or even 10 per centimetre (16 to 20 or even 24 per inch) – are used for this. The corners where three patches meet will be the weakest points, so it's a good idea to reinforce these with a few stitches.

This method is not suitable for fine fabrics such as silks, as they could be permanently marked by pins and needles. For these, secure the seam allowances with masking tape, and sew the corners through the seam allowances only.

Finishing

On completion press the patchwork on the wrong side and then pull out the basting threads (If you have avoided using back stitches, they will come out easily.) Press the right side if it needs it, protecting the surface with a cloth. Carefully lift out the papers.

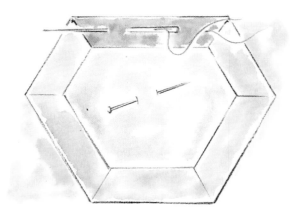

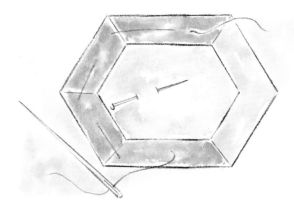

1 ♦ Pin a paper centrally to the wrong side of a fabric patch. Thread a needle but do not knot the end of the thread. Fold the material over one edge without creasing the paper. Holding it tightly, make the first basting stitch in the middle of the seam allowance, leaving the end of the thread free.

2 ♦ At each corner fold the material firmly over the point and put the needle through the fold to keep it in place. Repeat for the remaining edges.

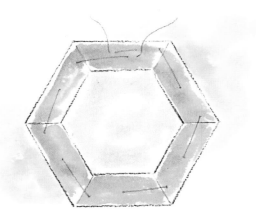

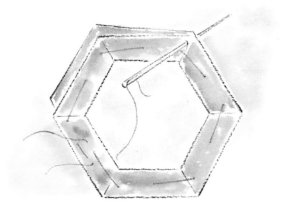

3 ♦ Do not make a backstitch at the end but overlap the beginning of the thread by one stitch. Leave the end free. By not fastening off this thread, you can easily remove it when the patchwork is complete. Press the patches gently before sewing them together to make the corners sharp.

4 ♦ To join two patches, place them right sides together with edges even and corners matching exactly. Insert the needle at a corner, under the fabric, and make a double stitch at the corner. Sew with very small, even, oversewing stitches to join the two edges. Press on the wrong side, then remove the basting.

HOLD IT!

This pretty pot holder, made entirely of hexagons,
offers a good chance to try English patchwork. Match the
fabrics to your kitchen colour scheme and it will not only be
functional but will brighten up your kitchen too.

SIZE

The pot holder is 28.6cm
(11¼ in) × 18.4cm (7¼ in).

YOU WILL NEED

25cm (¼ yd) each of 2 fabric
prints (A and B)

Matching threads

Small piece of wadding
(batting)

Stiff paper

Brass curtain ring

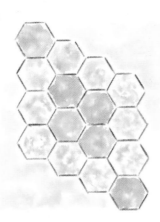

◆ *Assembly guide for honeycomb pot*
holder (make 2 – one for each side).

PREPARATION

Using the smaller template on
page 62–3, cut 32 hexagons from
paper.

Using the larger template on
pages 62–3, cut 12 hexagons from
print A and 20 from print B.

JOINING THE PATCHES

1 ◆ Make up 2 pieces of patchwork
fabric, each like the diagram
below, as instructed on page 35.
2 ◆ Press carefully on both the
wrong side and the right side.

MAKING UP

1 ◆ Cut a piece of wadding
(batting) the same shape as the
patchwork and baste it to the
wrong side of one piece.
2 ◆ Place the right side of this to
the right side of the remaining
piece of patchwork, and join the
edges by oversewing, leaving 2
sides of one hexagon open.
3 ◆ Turn right side out and push
out the point of each hexagon.
4 ◆ Remove all basting and papers
and join the 2 remaining sides of
the hexagon on the right side with
tiny stitches.
5 ◆ Press well. Sew on a brass ring
at one end for hanging.

HEXAGONAL TEMPLATES

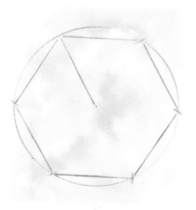

To make your own hexagonal
templates, set a compass to the
length you require each side to be,
and draw a circle. Keeping the
compass set to the same
measurement, place the compass
point anywhere on the circle and
mark the distance on the circle.
Move the compass point to that
mark and mark the distance again.
Continue around the circle until it
is divided into 6 equal segments.
Connect up the points with straight
lines to form a hexagon. Use this to
cut a template from stiff cardboard
or acetate.

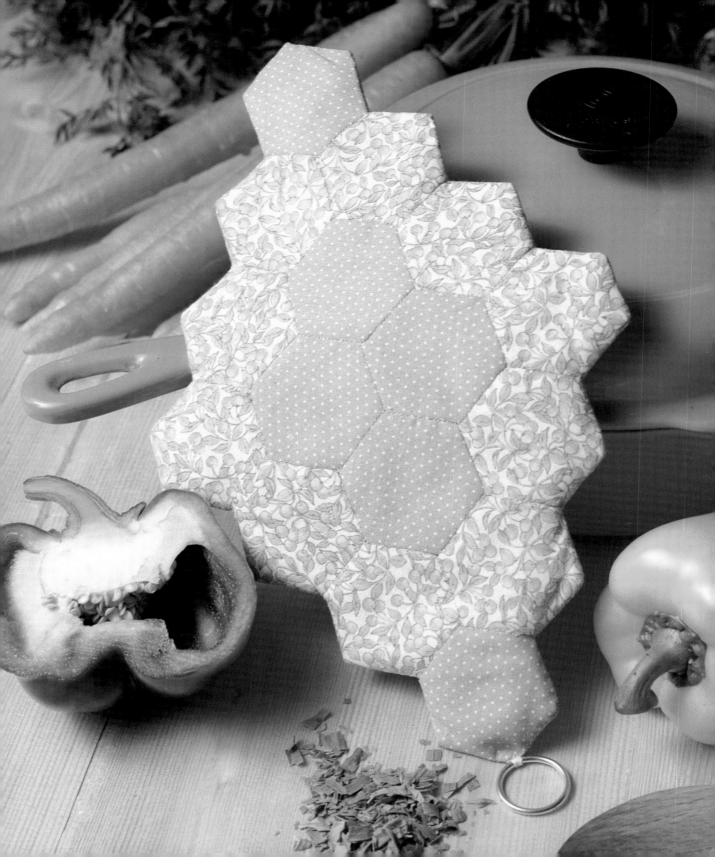

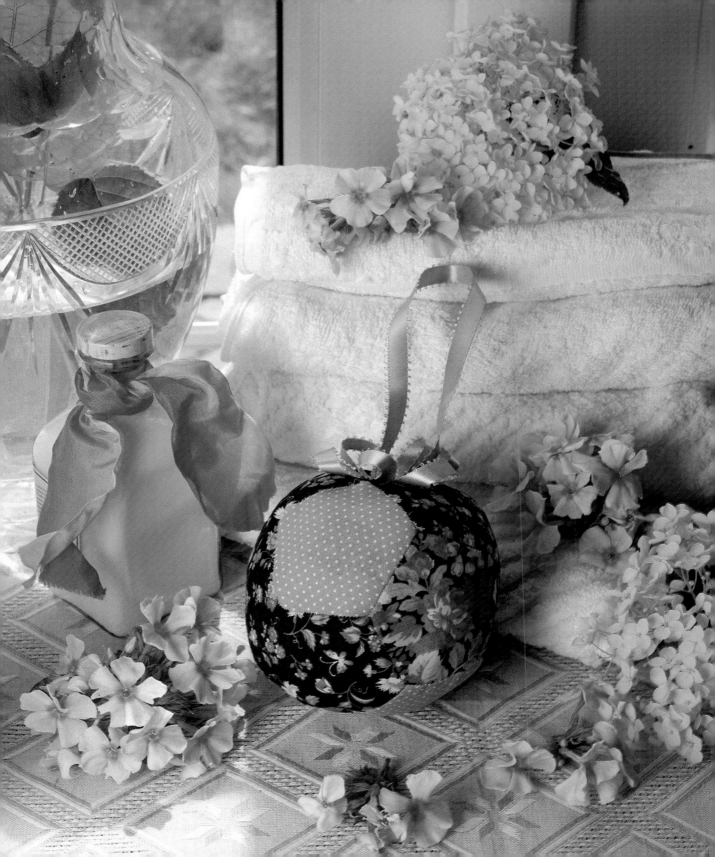

A NEW DIMENSION

Pentagons — five-sided shapes — are pieced over papers in much the same way as hexagons. As joined pentagons will not lie flat unless combined with other shapes, you can put this feature to good use by making a fragrant potpourri ball to hang in a cupboard.

SIZE

The potpourri ball is 10cm (4in) in diameter.

YOU WILL NEED

Scraps of fabric in 4 different prints

1m (1yd) of toning ribbon

Matching threads

Stiff paper

Wadding (batting)

Potpourri

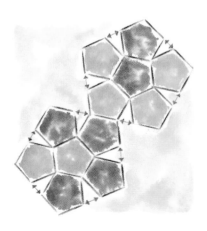

PREPARATION

Using the larger template on page 62–3, cut 12 fabric pentagons – 3 of each fabric design. Cut 12 papers using the smaller template.

JOINING THE PATCHES

1 ◆ Join the patches as described on page 35, following the diagram below, but leaving one side open.
2 ◆ Turn right side out and gently push out the corners of each shape.

MAKING UP

1 ◆ Half-fill the ball with the wadding (batting), place a handful of potpourri inside and then continue to stuff with wadding until a good round shape is achieved.
2 ◆ Remove the basting threads and papers, then close the seam on the outside, using tiny stitches.
3 ◆ Make a folded ribbon bow and sew it to the top of the ball, adding a longer piece for hanging.

◆ *Assembly guide for joining pentagon patches to make potpourri ball*

PENTAGON TEMPLATES

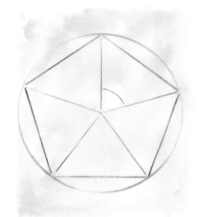

PENTAGON TEMPLATES

To draw a pentagon, you will need a protractor to measure the correct angle. First draw a circle, then draw a line from the centre of the circle to the edge. Using the protractor, measure an angle of exactly 72 degrees, drawing another line to the edge of the circle. Repeat this process 4 more times, and join up the 5 points with straight lines to form a pentagon. Use this to cut a template from stiff cardboard or acetate.

SUFFOLK PUFFS

Amazingly quick and easy to make, Suffolk Puffs can be used for bright and colourful items ranging from bedcovers and waistcoats to Christmas decorations and toys.

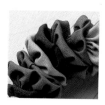

Originally developed in East Anglia, Suffolk Puffs are called Yorkshire Daisy in the north of England. They are also a traditional pattern in America, where they are known as Yo-Yos. But whichever name you prefer, this technique offers a fun way to try out patchwork without any longterm commitment of time. In fact, Suffolk Puffs are easy enough for a child to do.

Unlike the other types of patchwork in this book, Suffolk Puffs are purely decorative and do not join up to make a solid fabric. Although they can make an effective bedcover when used on their own, more usually the circles of material are gathered up, joined together and then mounted onto a coloured background fabric, which shows through the spaces between the puffs.

A simple, multi-coloured Suffolk Puff design will look attractive as a bedcover, or the puffs can be arranged in groups or blocks of colour. Another idea which can look very effective is to add print and plain puffs as borders on another piece of patchwork. You could even sew smaller ones on top of larger ones or embroider them with French knots or with a variety of cross stitches.

Suffolk Puffs can also be threaded through the middle with strong thread – or even with round elastic – to make delightful floppy toys. Being lightweight, they can also be used individually as whimsical Christmas tree decorations.

Cutting out the circles

To make the Suffolk Puffs you will need a number of fabric circles which are all the same size. It is best to use a circular template for this, which can be made very easily using a compass. Alternatively, if you don't have a compass, draw around a drinking glass, jar lid or small plate, depending on the size of circle you require. Remember to add a 6mm (¼ in) seam allowance all around.

The finished puff will be half the diameter of your circle, less 6mm (¼ in), so a 12.7cm (5in) circle of fabric will give you a 5.7cm (2¼ in) puff. It's a good idea to make the circles at least 6.3cm (2½ in).

A variety of fabrics can be used to make the Suffolk Puffs, but they should not be too bulky or you will have difficulty gathering them up. Cotton works well, but if you want to make an item for warmth, a very fine wool fabric can be used.

Whatever type of fabric you use, press it first and then lay the template on the fabric and draw around it with fade-away pen or pencil. Cut out the shapes accurately.

It is important to use a stronger than usual thread, such as the type of thread used for hand quilting. Traditionally the thread matches the fabric, but you could use contrasting thread instead if you prefer.

Padded puffs

As an alternative to the usual, flat Suffolk Puffs, you could stuff them with a lightweight wadding (batting). In this case, you will need another template, 6mm (¼ in) smaller than the size of the finished puffs. Use it to cut circles of polyester wadding. As you gather up the puffs, a circle of wadding can be enclosed in the centre if desired.

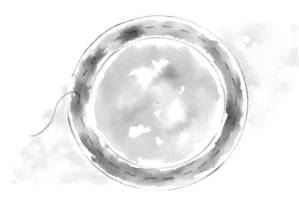

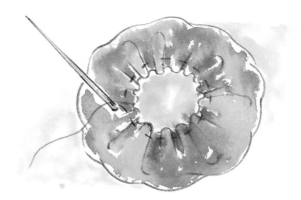

1 ◆ Turn your 6mm (¼ in) seam allowance to the wrong side all around the edge of the circle. Press or baste in place. Take a short length of strong thread and, using a double backstitch to begin, go around the circle through the turned hem with running stitches. Do not make the stitches too small or it will be difficult to gather the fabric.

2 ◆ Pull up the thread, gathering the fabric tightly into a circle. Fasten off very securely with a double backstitch through all layers of fabric to the back of the puff. Do not press.

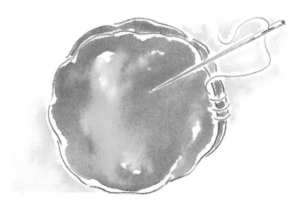

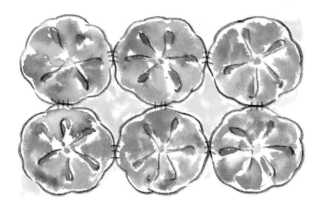

3 ◆ To join the puffs, place two of them together, gathered sides (the sides with the centre hole) facing each other. Using strong thread, make three small oversewing stitches at the edge of the two puffs, securing the ends firmly. Do not use more stitches than this or it could pull the circle out of shape. Fasten off the thread securely.

4 ◆ Suffolk Puffs can be joined together in the same way to form groups, each being stitched to its neighbour to form one piece. These can then be stitched to a backing fabric if required.

SWEET DREAMS

*Brighten up a baby's cradle or pram with this
cheerful quilt, which uses Suffolk Puff patchwork,
one of the quickest techniques of all. Made from cotton with a
polyester wadding (batting), it is fairly lightweight and
therefore ideal as a summer cover.*

SIZE

The quilt measures 86.4cm
(34in) × 62.5cm (24⅝ in).

YOU WILL NEED

1.4m (1½ yd) of white chintz
115cm (48in) wide

70cm (¾ yd) of red
patterned cotton 90cm (36in)
wide

62.5cm (⅝ yd) of green
patterned cotton 90cm (36in)
wide

50cm (½ yd) of blue
patterned cotton 90cm (36in)
wide

70cm (¾ yd) of wadding
(batting) 90cm (36in) wide

Strong thread in matching
colours

PREPARATION

Using the template on page 64,
cut the following circles: cut 34
from red patterned cotton, 26
from green patterned cotton and
17 from blue patterned cotton.

JOINING THE PATCHES

1 ◆ Turn 6mm (¼ in) of fabric to
the wrong side all around each
circle. Using matching thread,
make a double backstitch to start
and then work gathering stitches
around the turned-under edge.

2 ◆ Pull up tightly and fasten off
securely. Flatten each puff into a
circle with your fingers, but do not
press it.

3 ◆ When all the circles have been
gathered, join them up in the
pattern shown in the diagram on
this page. To join, place 2 Suffolk
Puffs together, with the gathered
sides facing and the flat sides
outside. Work 3 small oversewing
stitches, securing the ends firmly.

MAKING UP

1 ◆ When all the Suffolk Puffs have
been joined, cut a piece of white
chintz 2.5cm (1in) wider all
around than the completed
rectangle, and a piece of wadding
(batting) 10cm (4in) wider all
around.

2 ◆ Attach the puffs to the right
side of the white chintz by making
a few stitches through the centres.

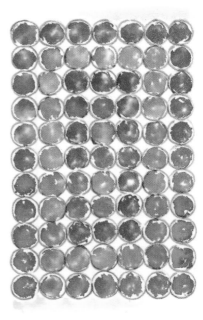

◆ *Colour pattern diagram showing the
arrangement of the three colours*

3 ◆ Stitch the wadding (batting)
to the back of the work 1.5cm
(⅝ in) from the edge by hand or
machine.

4 ◆ Cut a further piece of white
chintz 20cm (8in) wider all around
than before. With wrong sides

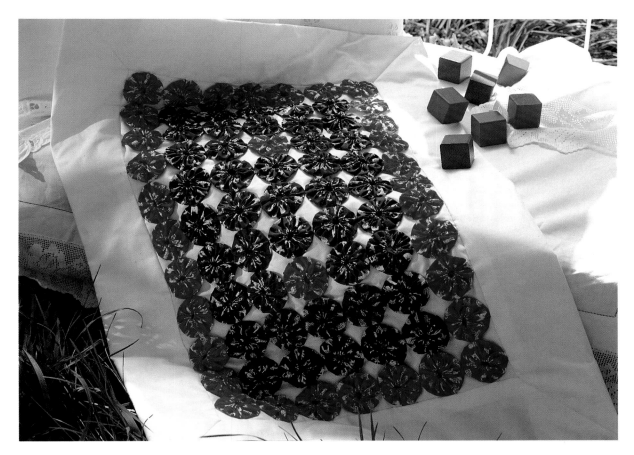

together, place the padded rectangle with puffs in the centre of this piece of fabric. Cut off a triangle of fabric from each corner to reduce the thickness.

5 ◆ Turn under about 2.5cm (1in) of fabric all around the edges and then fold the sides in to meet the edges of the puffs. Mitre the corners as shown in the diagrams. Hand sew along each side with small slip-stitches, catching in the edges of the puffs as you go along. Ladder-stitch (see page 68) the mitred corners.

6 ◆ Carefully press the quilt.

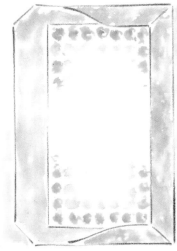

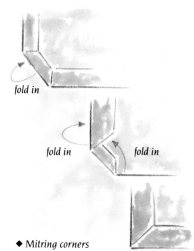

fold in

fold in   *fold in*

◆ *Mitring corners*

STRINGING ALONG

*This toy snake made from Suffolk Puffs strung
together looks and feels delightful. In a baby's nursery, however,
it should be kept out of reach, and for added safety the eyes
could simply be embroidered.*

SIZE

The snake is 35cm (14in) long.

YOU WILL NEED

Fabric in 5 shades of green (A, B, C, D and E)

Tiny scrap of red fabric

Matching strong thread

2 black sequins and 2 yellow beads, or tiny scraps of felt, or embroidery floss

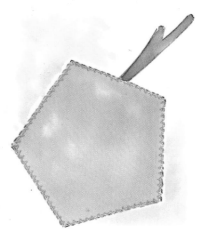

◆ *Zigzag stitching the snake's head*

PREPARATION

Using the templates on page 65, cut the following:

Pentagons: cut 2 from green shade E.

Triangles: cut 2 from green shade E.

Small circles: cut 2 from each of green shades, A, B, C and D.

Medium circles: cut 3 from each of green shades A, B, C and D plus 1 extra from any shade of green.

Large circles: cut 4 from each of green shades A, B, C and D.

Forked tongue shape: cut 1 from red fabric.

JOINING THE PATCHES

1 ◆ Make up the Suffolk Puffs as described on page 41, turning under 6mm (¼ in) all around each circle and gathering with the strong thread. Pull up the gathers and fasten off very firmly. Continue until all 37 circles have been gathered.

2 ◆ Join the triangles by zigzag stitching on the sewing machine. Zigzag stitch around the edges of the tongue shape.

3 ◆ Place the 2 pentagons with right sides together, and, using a straight stitch, machine around 4 of the 5 sides, taking a 6mm (¼ in) seam. Turn right side out.

4 ◆ Place the tongue shape in the centre of the remaining side of the pentagon. Baste in place and then zigzag stitch all around the pentagon in green thread, catching in the tongue as you stitch.

5 ◆ Sew on sequins with a bead in the centre of each for eyes. If, however, the toy is for a young child, use scraps of felt for the eyes or embroider them.

MAKING UP

1 ◆ Thread your needle with 2 lengths of thread and double these so that you have 4 threads. Attach this securely by oversewing to the centre of the short side of the triangle.

2 ◆ Thread 8 small puffs onto the thread, followed by 8 medium puffs, 16 large ones and finally 5 more medium ones.

3 ◆ Fasten the string of Suffolk Puffs to the end of the head pentagon with several strong oversewing stitches in the centre.

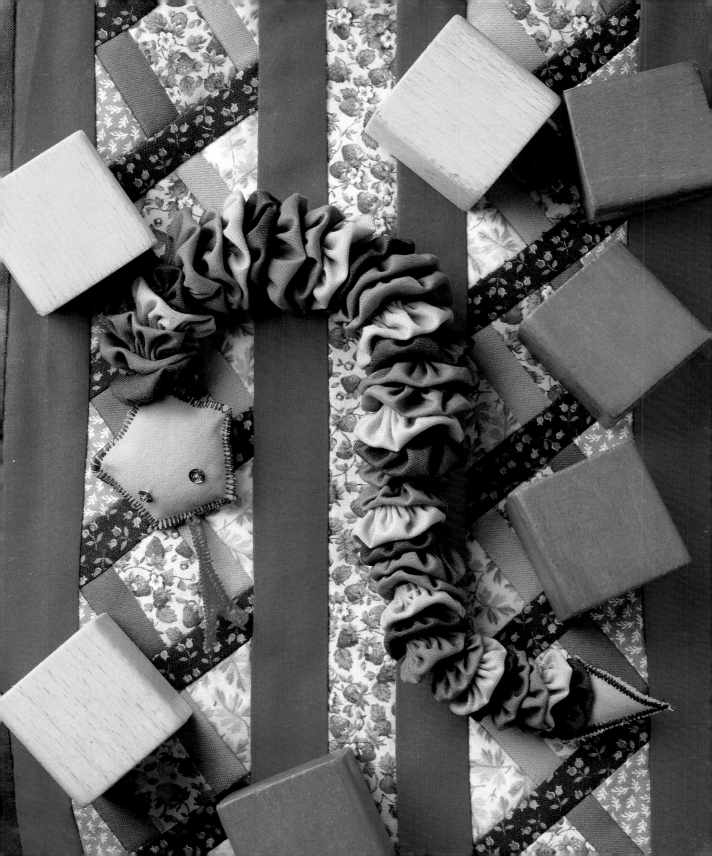

LOG CABIN PATCHWORK

*Possibly the oldest form of patchwork, Log Cabin
is also the best-known. Practical as well as decorative,
it produces a strong fabric and is a useful way of using up
narrow strips of leftover material.*

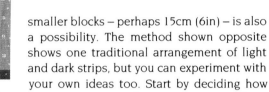

Log Cabin involves sewing strips of fabric straight onto a background fabric rather than joining the strips to each other as in most other forms of patchwork. The strips, which are grouped into light and dark colours, surround a small central square to form a larger square. The squares, or 'blocks' (see page 16), are then joined to form a design.

Symbolism of the pattern

Although Log Cabin was popular in the 18th and 19th centuries in Britain as well as in North America, it takes its name from the resemblance of the strips to the logs of the cabins built by the settlers in the New World.

The central square, which was traditionally red, is believed to have represented firelight, which created light areas and shadows in the log cabins. When completed, the blocks can be arranged, or 'set', in a variety of ways to produce further patterns, with intriguing names like Straight Furrow, Barn Raising and Windmill Blades. The blocks themselves may also have a variety of different arrangements of light and dark strips.

Building up a design

Calico (muslin in the United States) is an ideal backing fabric. A good size for the backing square of a large article is 30cm (12in); squares can then be joined to form a piece as large as is required. Alternatively, a single square can be used on its own for, say, a cushion cover or tablemat. A combination of

smaller blocks – perhaps 15cm (6in) – is also a possibility. The method shown opposite shows one traditional arrangement of light and dark strips, but you can experiment with your own ideas too. Start by deciding how wide you want your strips to be – 2.5cm (1in) is about average – then add 6mm (¼ in) on each side for the seam allowance.

The central square of fabric is usually twice the width of the strips, so if you are using 2.5cm (1in) strips (excluding the seam allowances), the square will need to be 5cm (2in) wide. Again, you need to add a 6mm (¼ in) seam allowance.

If you draw a pattern on a square of paper the same size as your backing square, you can determine the length of each fabric strip needed. In each new round, the strips will need to be 5cm (2in) longer than the four from the previous round. Cut all strips on the straight grain.

Using light and dark

You will need equal quantities of light and dark fabric, because each 'round' of strips around the central fabric square is made up of two light and two dark strips. Avoid using medium tones, as this would dilute the effect. The central square can actually be any colour unless you wish to opt for the traditional red used in the original log cabin quilts.

Always start on the same side of the square, using two light and two dark strips on every round. The edges of the final strips should be even with the edges of the backing square.

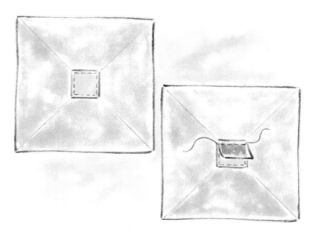

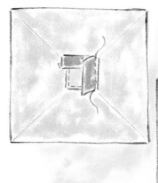

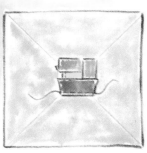

1 ◆ On the backing square, mark the diagonals with fade-away pen or pencil or basting stitches to help with the placing of the pieces. Cut a 5cm (2in) square for the centre and place it on the backing square, stitching all around. Now, with right sides facing, place the first light strip on the centre square, with raw edges even, and stitch 6mm (¼ in) from the edge, through all layers. Open it out so the right side is on top; press flat.

2 ◆ Attach the second light strip in the same way, placing it along the adjacent edge of the square, with the end over the end of the first strip. After stitching, fold back and press. Add the third strip, this time in dark fabric, in the same way.

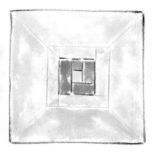

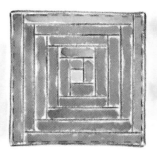

3 ◆ Now add the fourth strip, which should again be dark, to complete the round. The diagram above shows the order in which a round is worked. Continue in this way, covering the raw edges of the first row of strips with the next round, and so gradually building up the square.

4 ◆ Baste around the raw edges of the final strip and the backing square to ensure a flat finish when joining blocks. Finally, sew the completed blocks together to form pieced strips, then join the strips.

FAIR AND SQUARE

Log Cabin patchwork is ideal for a tote bag like this because the backing fabric to which the strips are sewn makes it sturdy, and the traditional arrangement of light and dark strips bordering a square adds visual interest.

SIZE

The bag measures 35.5cm (14in) × 56cm (22in).

YOU WILL NEED

1.2m (1¼ yd) of calico (muslin in the U.S.)

1m (1yd) of plain fabric

35cm (⅜ yd) each of 6 dark print and 6 light print fabrics

Matching thread

56cm (22in) zip

2.9m (3⅛ yd) of woven webbing

Piece of strong cardboard 17.8cm (7in) × 56cm (22in)

PREPARATION

1 ◆ Using the 2 pattern pieces on pages 58–9, cut one main bag piece from calico (muslin in the United States). The calico is folded in half and each half is used as a backing square for each long side of the bag.
2 ◆ Cut 2 pieces for the ends of the bag from calico and 2 from the plain fabric. Transfer markings.

3 ◆ Using the template on page 66, cut 2 squares from one of the light-coloured prints.
4 ◆ Cut four 5cm (2in) × 20cm (8in) strips from another light-coloured print and 4 from a dark print. Continue to cut 4 light strips and 4 dark strips for each round, making the strips for each new round 5cm (2in) longer than those in the previous round. In the end you should have 24 light strips and 24 dark strips in graduated lengths.

JOINING THE PATCHES

1 ◆ Fold the calico backing in half as shown. Using your ruler and a pencil, mark diagonal lines on this foundation fabric from both top corners to the corners diagonally opposite, crossing in the centre. Add the horizontal and vertical lines, which also go through the centre. These will help with the placing of the fabric strips.
2 ◆ Position the fabric square exactly in the centre of the calico, using the pencil lines for guidance; baste in place.
3 ◆ Now place the shortest of your light strips of fabric right side down on the calico so that one

long edge is even with one edge of the central square. Stitch 6mm (¼ in) from the edge. Fold the strip back and press carefully.
4 ◆ Sew the second strip of light fabric along the second side of the central square, overlapping the first strip at the end. Once again fold back and press.
5 ◆ Now take a dark strip of the same length and continue along the next side of the square, overlapping as before. Fold back and press.
6 ◆ The fourth strip, again a dark one, is added to the remaining side of the original square, overlapping the first and third strips at the ends. Fold back and press. This completes the first round.

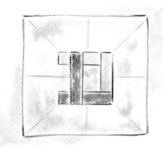

◆ *Stitching on the fourth strip in the first round of the block*

7 ◆ Repeat steps 1–6 on the other half of the calico for the second side of the bag.

8 ◆ For the second round, start on the same side as in the previous round with a light strip of the next length, then another light strip, followed by two dark strips. Duplicate this on the other half.

9 ◆ Continue in the same way until all the strips are used and the calico is covered.

MAKING UP

1 ◆ Cut a piece of webbing 2.8m (110 in) long. Put a pin in the webbing 42cm (16½ in) from one end, and another pin 56cm (22in) from the first. Form a circle with the webbing and join the ends together with the zigzag stitch.

2 ◆ Using the pins as guides, place the joined ends of the webbing on the stars at one end of the bag. Pin the centre of the remaining webbing along the guidelines marked on the bag.

3 ◆ Stitch the webbing in place between the stars close to the long edges. At each star, form a box with your stitches which is the width of the webbing, and

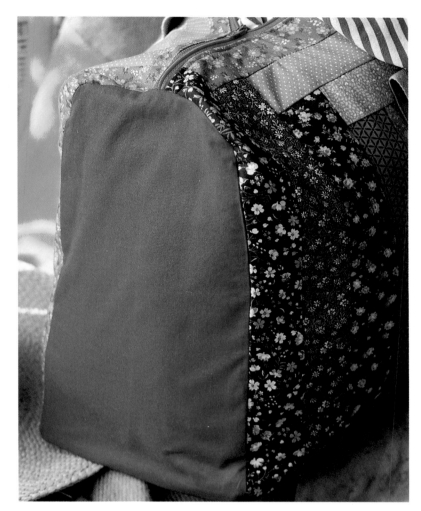

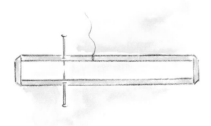

◆ *Forming webbing into circle after marking with pins at appropriate points*

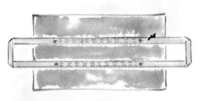

◆ *Centring webbing on placement lines and stitching between stars close to edges*

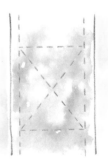

◆ *Stitching webbing to reinforce points marked with stars*

stitch across the diagonals for reinforcement.

4 ◆ Open the zip and place it face down on the right side of the seam allowance along the upper edge on one side of the bag. Position the end of the zip at the large O, centring the zip tape over the seamline.

5 ◆ Baste in place, then stitch, being careful to stitch in the centre of the zip tape while keeping the bag free. Repeat for the other side of the zip.

6 ◆ Press the zip tape towards the bag, turning the teeth out. Edge-stitch the bag along each side of the zip as shown.

7 ◆ Place one calico endpiece and one plain endpiece together with wrong sides facing. Baste all around. Do the same with the other 2 pieces.

8 ◆ With right sides together, pin each end section to the sides of the bag, matching the marked points and clipping the bag at intervals if necessary.

9 ◆ Stitch all around, taking a 1.5cm (⅝ in) seam. Stitch again several times at each end of the zip to reinforce it. Trim the seams and zigzag stitch the edges to neaten them. Turn the bag right side out and press carefully.

10 ◆ Cut a piece of plain fabric 59cm (23¼ in) × 38.7cm (15¼ in). Fold this in half crosswise and place the piece of cardboard inside; turn 1.5cm (⅝ in) under on all 3 sides of both halves. Stitch close to the edge, enclosing the cardboard. Place the covered cardboard inside the bag to form a rigid base.

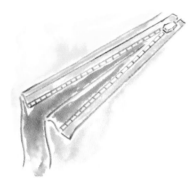

◆ *Inserting zip*

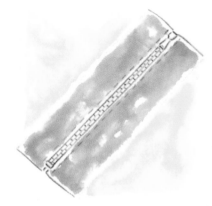

◆ *Edge-stitching alongside zip on right side*

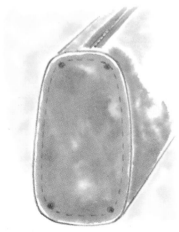

◆ *Stitching end sections to each side of bag*

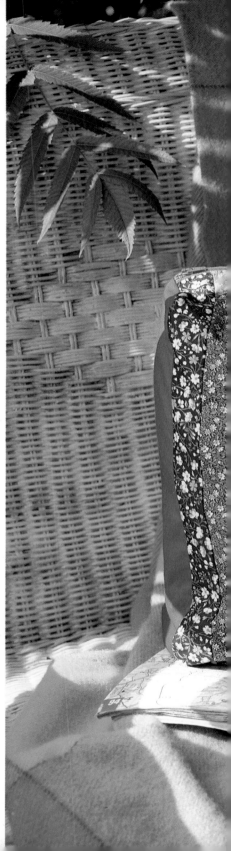

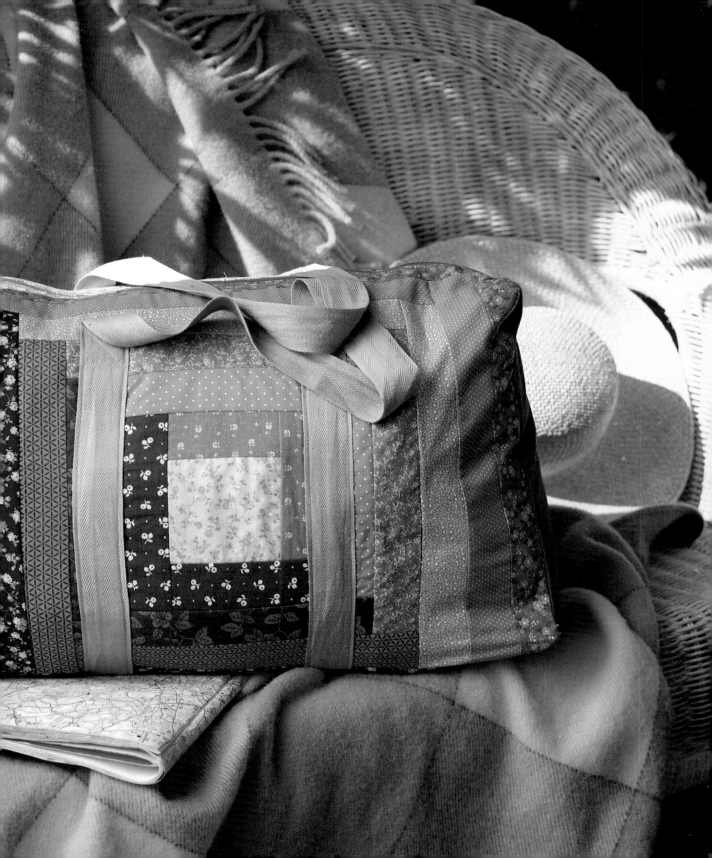

Cathedral Window Patchwork

*Another technique that is dramatically easier
than it looks, Cathedral Window patchwork is based
on the folding and refolding of fabric squares to create a
stained-glass window effect.*

The Cathedral Window technique is also known as Mayflower patchwork, as it is said to have been developed by the Pilgrims who travelled from England to North America in the early 17th century in the *Mayflower*. It is an extremely practical form of patchwork because the foundation fabric itself forms a neat backing and edging. And, although it has no other backing or any padding, the many layers of fabric that are involved make it surprisingly warm.

With this technique, plain squares are folded, refolded and sewn together. Smaller squares, in a contrasting fabric, are then sewn over the 'window frames' formed by the plain squares. The 'frames' are curved around the 'windows' by rolling the folded edges over the raw edges of the contrasting fabric and are then sewn in place invisibly. When deciding the size of a design, bear in mind that the twice-folded squares will be only half their original size. The squares you cut, therefore, ought to be at least 15.2cm (6in).

At the edges of a piece of Cathedral Window patchwork you will have half-squares (ie triangles). These can be left blank if you wish, or the pattern can be continued to the edge by making more half-squares as shown opposite (step 5).

Choose fabrics that do not require ironing after being washed, to avoid crushing the folds.

MAKING CATHEDRAL WINDOWS

1 ◆ Cut a 15.2cm (6in) square from the main fabric, on the straight grain. Mark the centre point of the square on the wrong side. Turn a 6mm (¼ in) hem to the wrong side on all four edges, and baste or press down. Fold each point of the square to the marked centre and pin in place. Press.

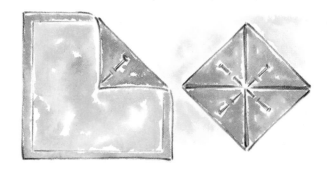

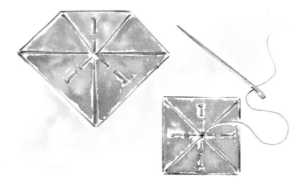

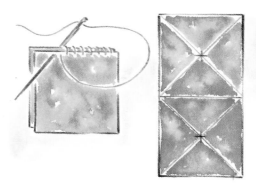

2 ◆ Now fold each new point to the centre, pinning in place and removing the pins from the first layer as you go. Sew the points of the square into the centre with a double thickness of matching thread, using tiny stitches through all the layers of fabric.

3 ◆ Repeat this with another square the same size, then place the folded sides of two squares together and oversew with tiny, neat stitches along one edge of the square. Open out and press.

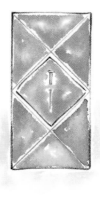

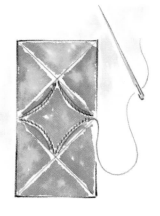

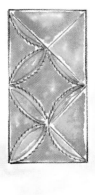

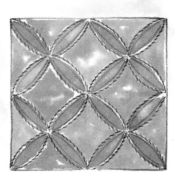

4 ◆ Cut a square of contrasting fabric a fraction smaller than the diagonal square formed by the joined folded squares. Place this right-side-up in the centre and pin it in position. Take the folded edge running alongside the raw edge of the small square on one side and roll it over the raw edge. Sew the folded edge in place using small, invisible running stitches or slip-stitch, making sure that all the raw edge is completely covered. It should taper to a point at each end. Repeat this process on the other three sides of the square, sewing them together neatly at the corners.

5 ◆ If you want to continue the pattern to the edge, take another small square in the contrast fabric and fold it in half diagonally. Draw a line 6mm (¼ in) below the halfway line, and cut off this smaller triangle beyond it. Turn the seam allowance to the wrong side and press or baste. Position the contrasting triangle in the half-square and sew in place as before by rolling the folded edges over the raw edges. Oversew the turned edge and the folded edge of the large square together.

Rainbow Colours

Enhance the stained-glass effect of Cathedral Window patchwork by using shining silks and ribbons in wonderful vivid colours to make this beautiful cushion.

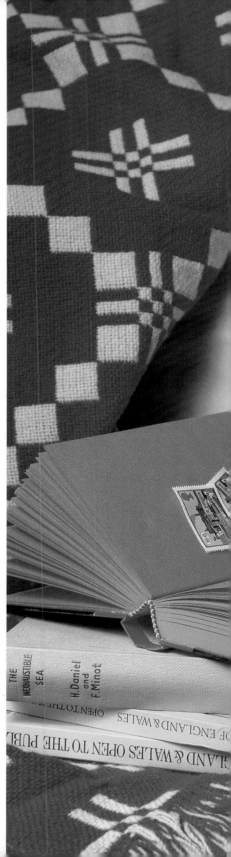

SIZE

The cushion measures 34cm (13½ in) square.

YOU WILL NEED

1.25m (1⅜ yd) of fuchsia silk

10cm (⅛ yd) each of yellow, purple, blue, magenta and red silk

Matching silk thread

Zip

1.9m (2yd) of piping cord (optional)

1.9m (2yd) of ribbon at least 3mm (⅛ in) wide in same colours as silk

Cushion pad measuring 34cm (13½ in) square

PREPARATION

Using the templates on page 67, cut the following squares.

15.2cm (6in) squares: cut 25 from fuchsia pink silk

4.5cm (1¾ in) squares: cut 6 from magenta, 8 each from blue, purple and yellow, and 10 from red silk.

JOINING THE PATCHES

1 ◆ Assemble the fuchsia background squares as described on page 52–3, steps 1–4.

2 ◆ Add smaller squares as shown in the pattern diagram overleaf. If you are using other colours or would like to try a different layout with your colours, simply draw a grid and use coloured felt-tip pens to experiment.

3 ◆ You will finish up with a piece of patchwork fabric which is 5 squares by 5 squares.

MAKING UP

1 ◆ Measure the patchwork fabric and cut a further piece of the fuchsia background fabric to these dimensions plus an extra 6.3cm (2½ in) on the width and an extra 3.2cm (1¼ in) on the length. Fold this piece in half crosswise and cut it into 2 pieces along the fold.

2 ◆ Taking a 1.5cm (⅝ in) seam, baste the 2 pieces together. Stitch the seam, leaving an opening in the centre the length of your zip. Insert the zip using the zipper foot on your machine. Open the zip. If you are not planning to pipe the edge of the cushion, skip steps 3, 4 and 7.

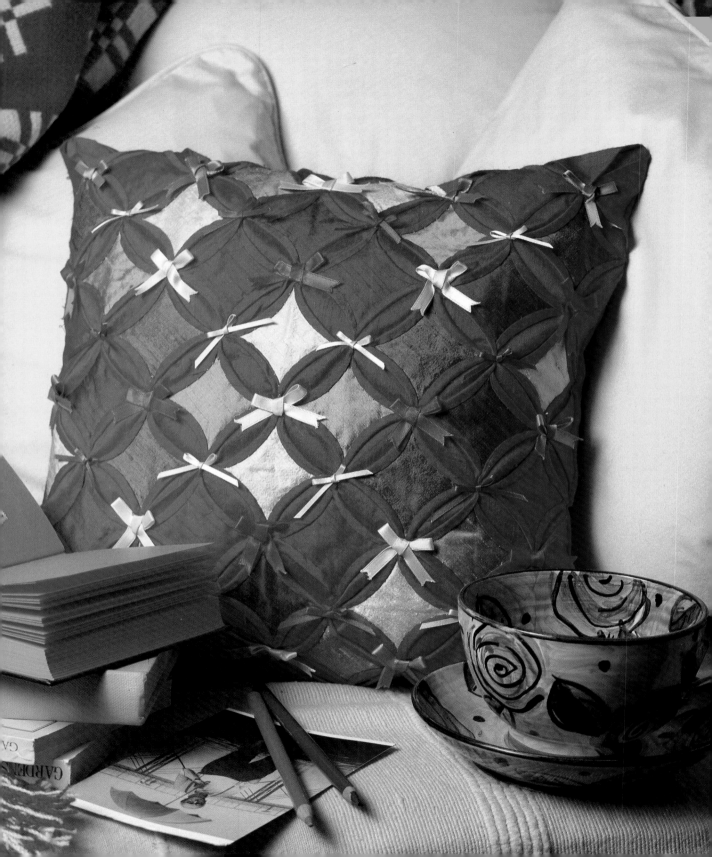

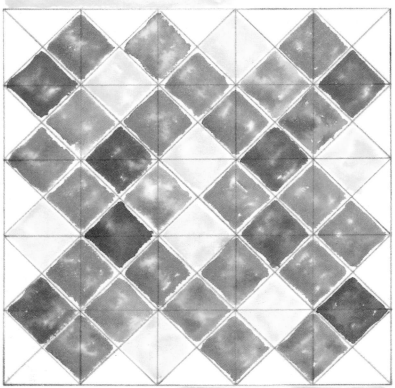

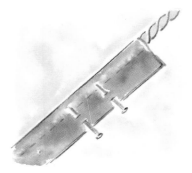

◆ Measuring fabric to cover piping cord

◆ Stitching fabric over cord

3 ◆ If you *are* planning to pipe it, fold a corner of the fabric over the piping cord; pin, encasing the cord snugly. Measure 1.5cm (⅝ in) out from the pin, and mark this point. Unpin and unfold. This will tell you the width of fabric strips you'll need to cut in order to cover the cord. Cut enough strips of this width in your chosen fabric to go all around your cushion. Cut them on the bias, joining the strips as necessary to give the required length.

4 ◆ Wrap the strip around the cord with the fabric right side out and edges even. With the zipper foot on the machine, stitch close to the cord, using a long straight stitch and stretching the cord as you sew.

5 ◆ Pin the covered cord to the edge of your patchwork piece with the raw edges even and the cord towards the centre. Baste carefully in place.

6 ◆ Place the backing piece and the patchwork piece together, right sides facing. With the zipper foot still on the machine, baste through all layers all around the seamline, taking a 1.5cm (⅝ in)

seam and clipping into the seam allowance at the corners. Stitch the seam.

7 ◆ Trim the ends of the piping cord and sew them together by hand. Overlap the ends of the fabric strip, turning under the raw edge on top by 6mm (¼ in).

8 ◆ Turn the cushion cover right side out but do not press as this would spoil the effect of the patchwork.

9 ◆ Make small bows with the ribbon and sew on one at the point of each square. Insert the cushion pad.

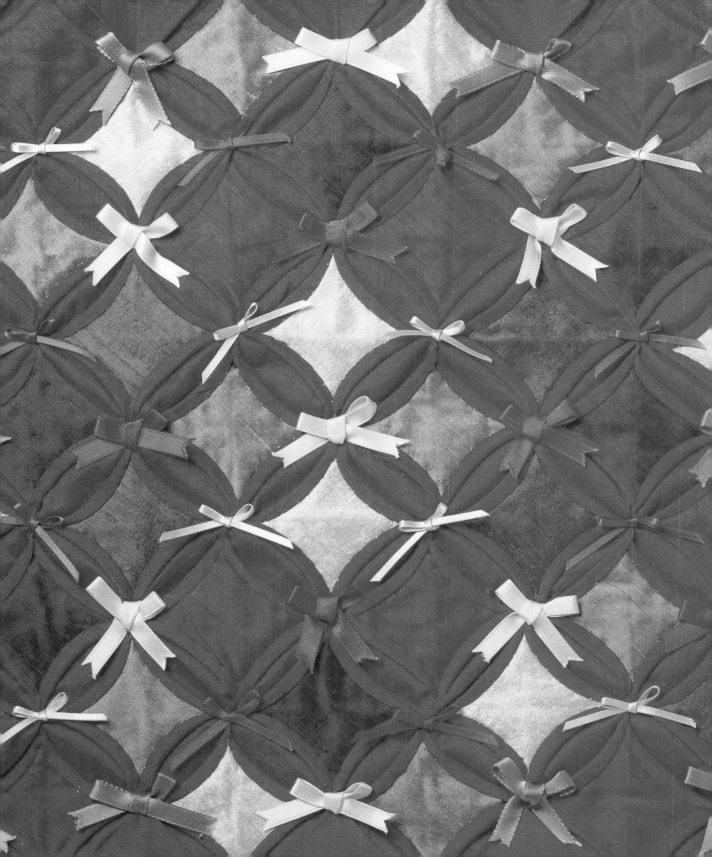

Patterns

Use these patterns to complete the
Seminole patchwork cafetière cover on page 24 and the Log Cabin
patchwork tote bag on page 48.

Enlarge with a photocopier or by copying onto a grid; each square = 5cm (2in).

CAFETIÈRE COVER	**TOTE BAG**
pages 24–5	*pages 48–51*

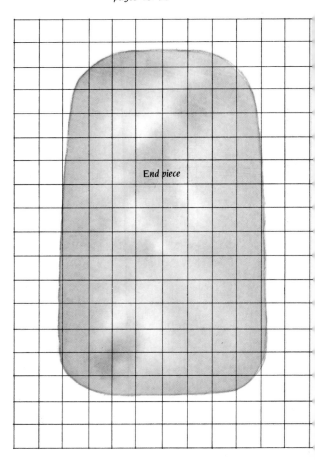

End piece

Main piece

TEMPLATES

*These templates are all full size. Photostat or
trace them, transfer the lines to stiff cardboard and
then cut them out. When using them, follow the instructions
for each project.*

CURTAINS

pages 14–15

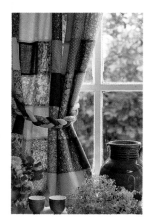

pages 18–21

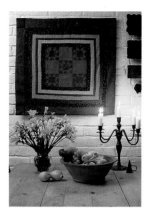

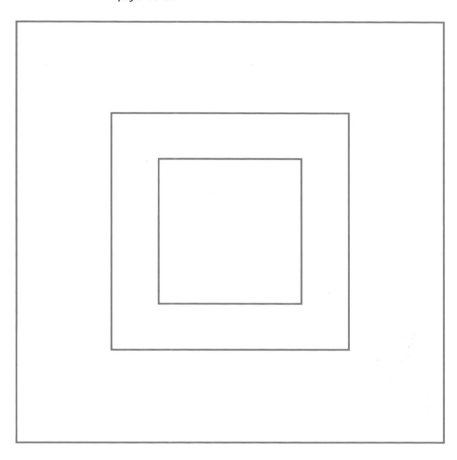

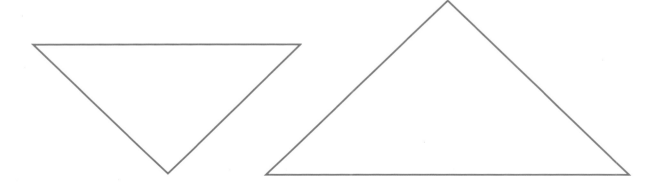

GREETINGS CARDS

pages 30–1

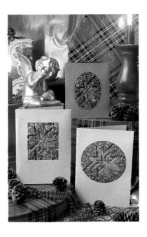

TRINKET BOX AND BROOCH

pages 32–3

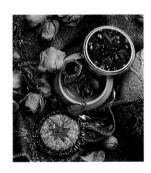

POT HOLDER

pages 36–7

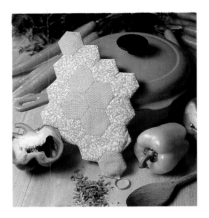

POTPOURRI BALL

pages 38–9

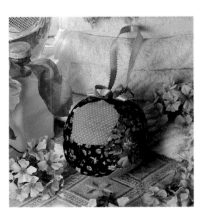

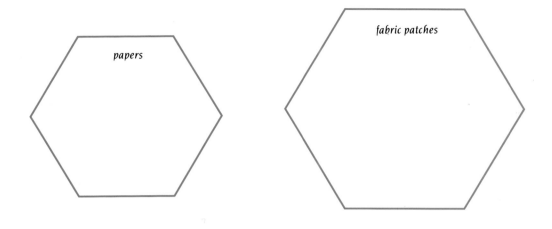

papers

fabric patches

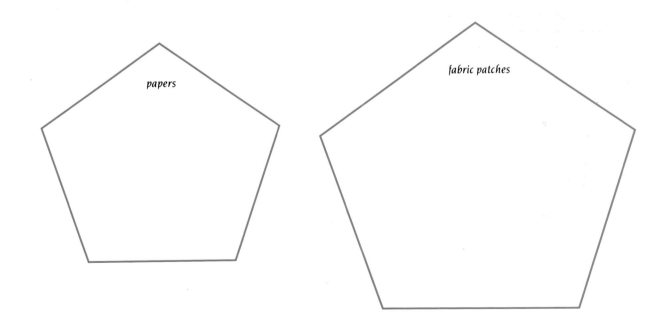

papers

fabric patches

pages 42–3

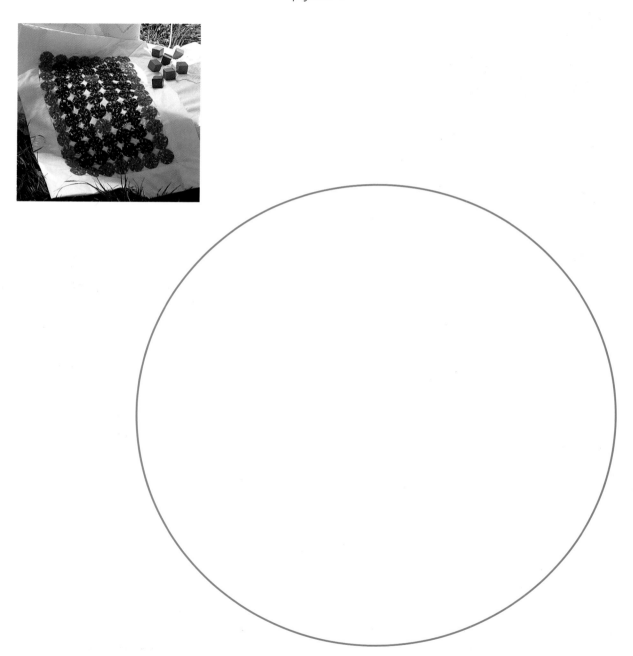

pages 44–5

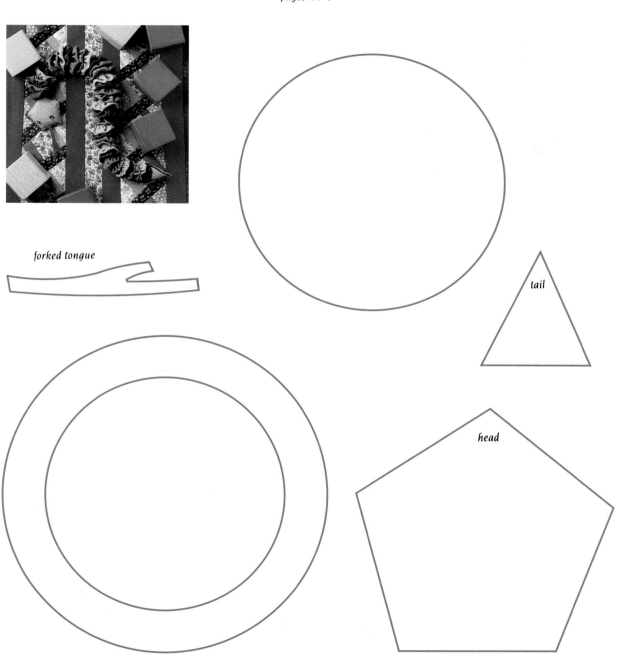

forked tongue

tail

head

TOTE BAG

pages 48–50

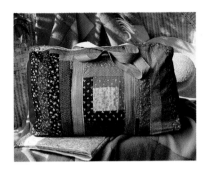

CUSHION

pages 54–7

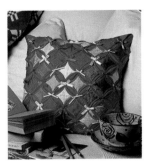

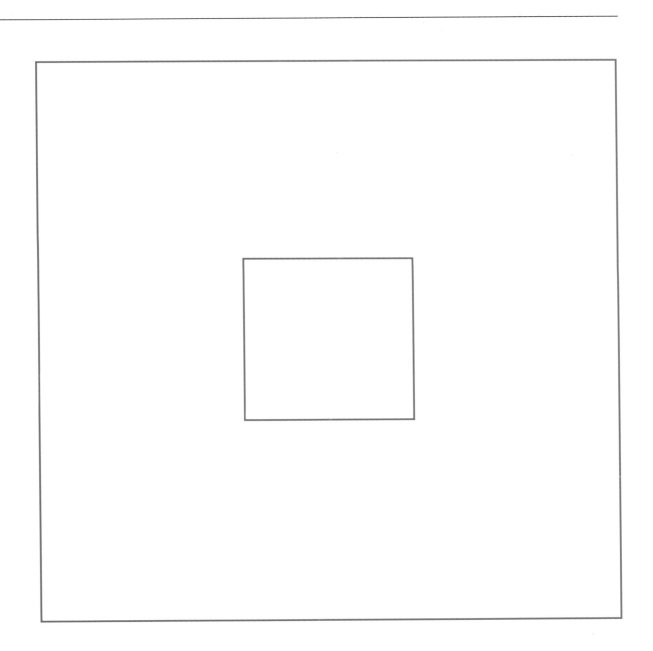

HAND STITCHES

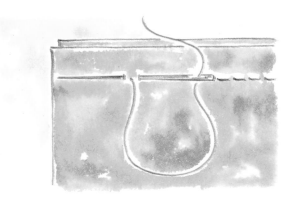

BACKSTITCH
Use this stitch to begin or end in hand sewing. Working from right to left and keeping stitches very small, bring the needle through the fabric from the underside, then take a stitch one stitch-length behind and bring it out a double stitch-length ahead. Pull the thread through.

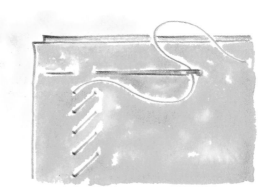

DIAGONAL BASTING
Use this to hold fabric layers flat together during making up. It is particularly useful when inserting wadding (batting) and it covers large areas quickly. Make small, evenly spaced stitches parallel to one another and at right angles to the edge by putting the needle in from right to left. Do not pull the thread tight or ridges will appear. On the upper side this will make diagonal stitches and on the underside horizontal stitches.

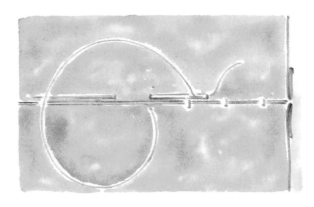

LADDER STITCH
This is a variation of slip-stitch, which is used to join two folded edges together. Thread the needle along inside the fold on each side, giving an invisible join.

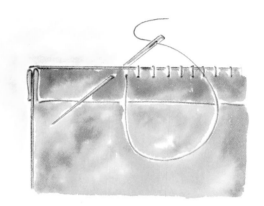

OVERSEWING (OVERHAND STITCH)

Use this to join two finished edges. Insert the needle diagonally from the back edge through the front edge, picking up one or two threads at a time. Insert the needle immediately behind the thread from the previous stitch and bring it out a stitch-length away. Keep all your stitches the same size and distance apart; they should be tiny, straight and even.

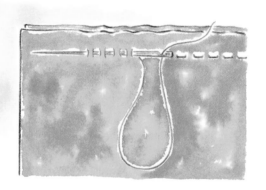

RUNNING STITCH

This stitch has many uses, including seams not requiring much strength, and gathering. Working from right to left, weave the point of the needle in and out of the fabric several times then pull the thread through. Keep the stitches the same size and evenly spaced apart.

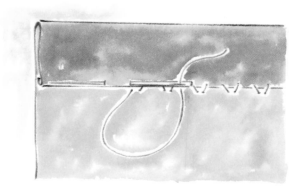

SLIP-STITCH

Use this nearly invisible stitch to join a folded edge to a flat surface. Working from right to left, fasten the thread and bring the needle through the folded edge. Pick up one or two threads of the under-fabric. Slip the needle through the folded fabric for about 3–6 mm (⅛–¼ inches). Bring the needle out and pick up another one or two stitches of the under-fabric.

INDEX

ACKNOWLEDGEMENTS

The author would like to thank the following suppliers for their assistance; all operate a mail order service.
Strawberry Fayre, Chagford, Devon TQ13 8EN, for fabric for curtains, place mat, cafetière cover, snake, potpourri ball, potholder and cards.
Village Fabrics, PO Box 43, Wallingford, Oxfordshire OX10 9DF, for fabrics for pram cover, wall hanging, trinket box lid and brooch.
Framecraft Miniatures Ltd, 148-150 High Street, Aston, Birmingham B6 4US, for trinket box and brooch mount.
James Hare Ltd, PO Box 72, Queen Street, Leeds LS1 1XL, for fabrics for silk cushion cover.
Mulberry Silks, Old Rectory Cottage, Easton Grey, Malmesbury, Wiltshire SN16 0PE, for silk threads.

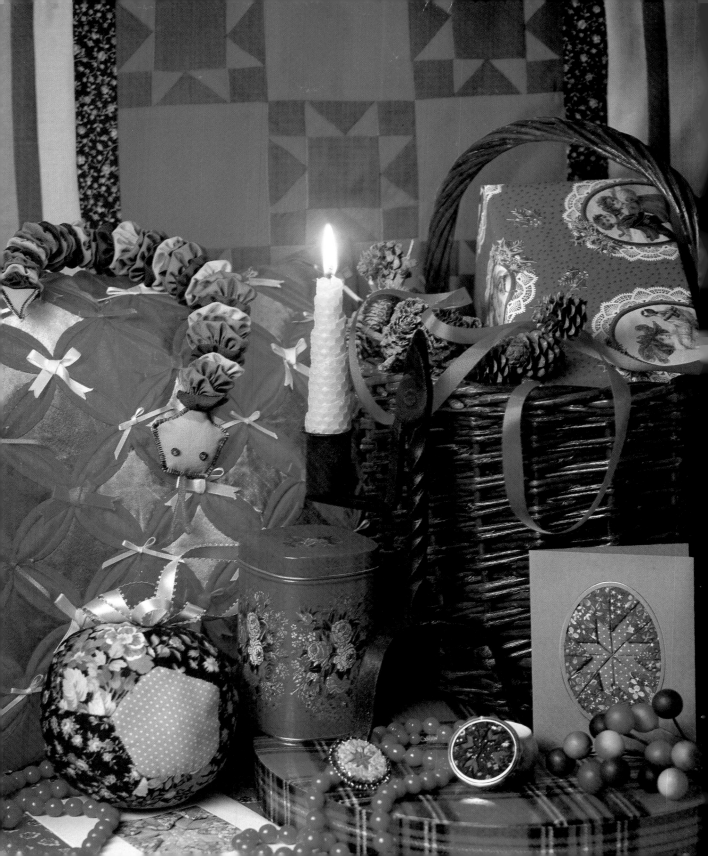

Take up
PATCHWORK

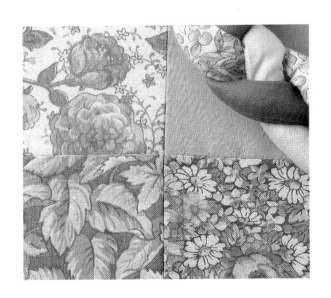

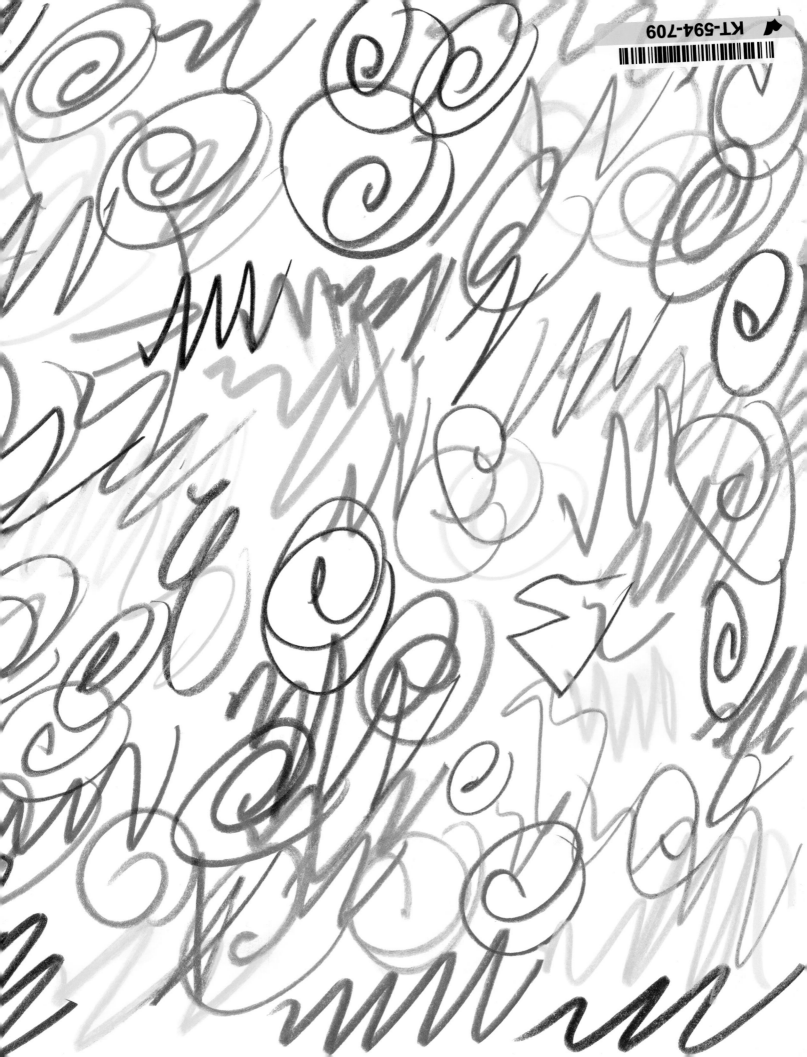

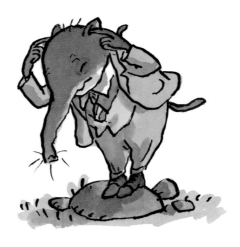

This paperback edition first published in 2006 by Andersen Press Ltd.
The rights of Jeanne Willis and Tony Ross to be identified as the author and illustrator of this
work have been asserted by them in accordance with the Copyright, Designs and Patents Act, 1988.
First published in Great Britain in 2004 by Andersen Press Ltd., 20 Vauxhall Bridge Road, London SW1V 2SA.
Published in Australia by Random House Australia Pty., 20 Alfred Street, Milsons Point, Sydney, NSW 2061.
All rights reserved. Colour separated in Switzerland by Photolitho AG, Zürich.
Printed and bound in Singapore.

10   9   8   7   6   5   4   3   2   1

British Library Cataloguing in Publication Data available.

ISBN-10:1 84270 566 0
ISBN-13: 978 184270 566 7

This book has been printed on acid-free paper

Shhh!

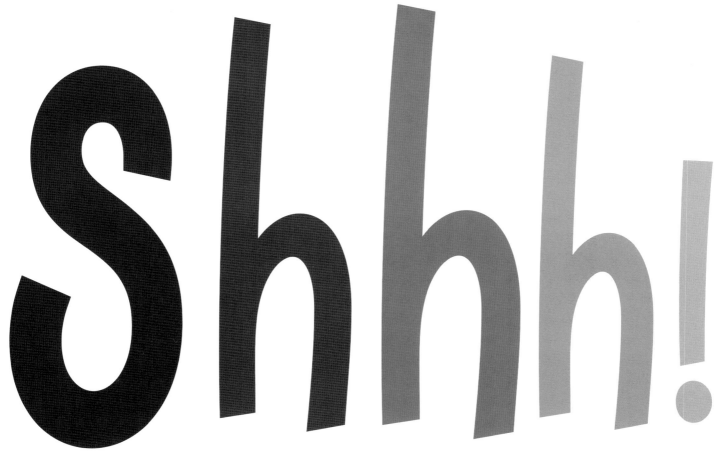

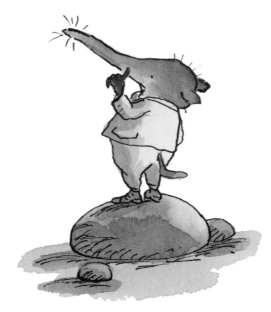

Jeanne Willis   Tony Ross

Andersen Press
London

A little shrew had wonderful news!
He wanted to tell the whole world,
But it was too noisy:

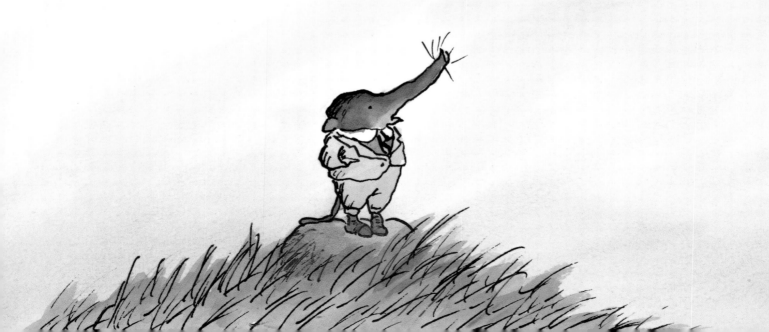

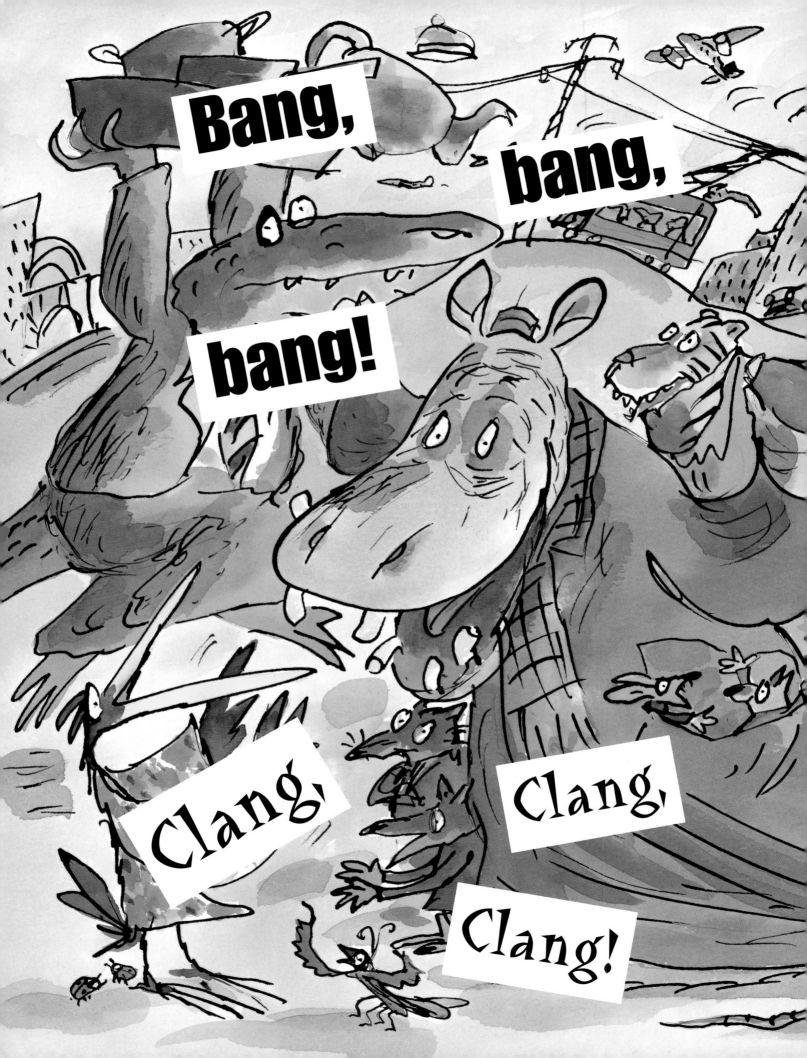

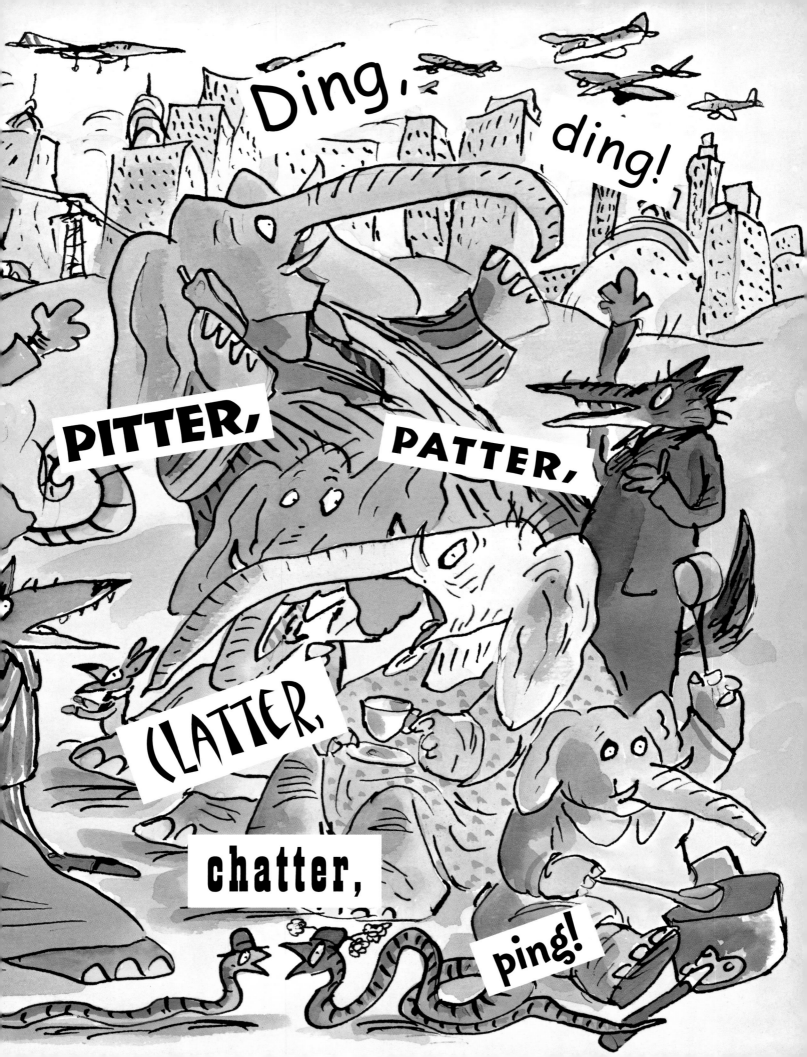

The shrew had a great big thing to say.

But he only had a very small voice.

No one could hear him above the noise:

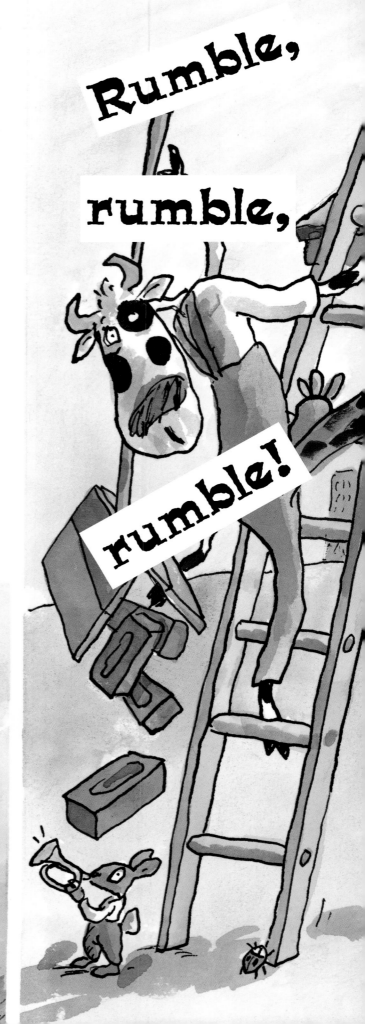

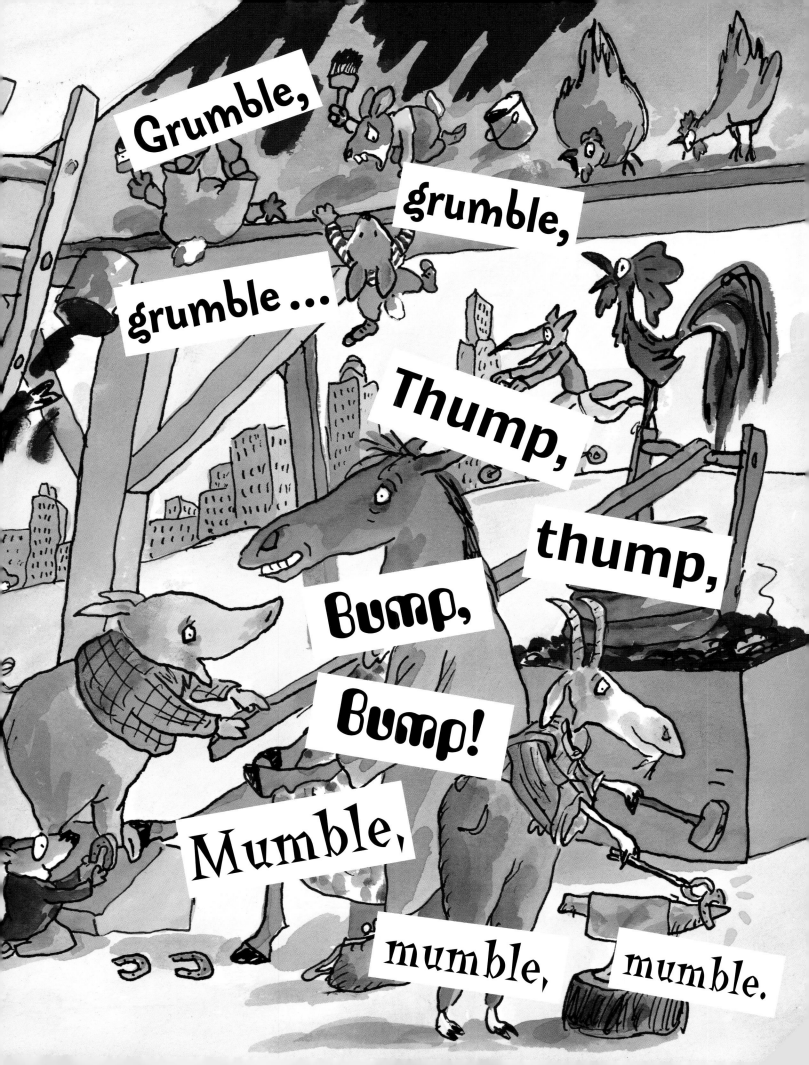

The shrew waited all day.

He waited all night for quiet.

But it never came:

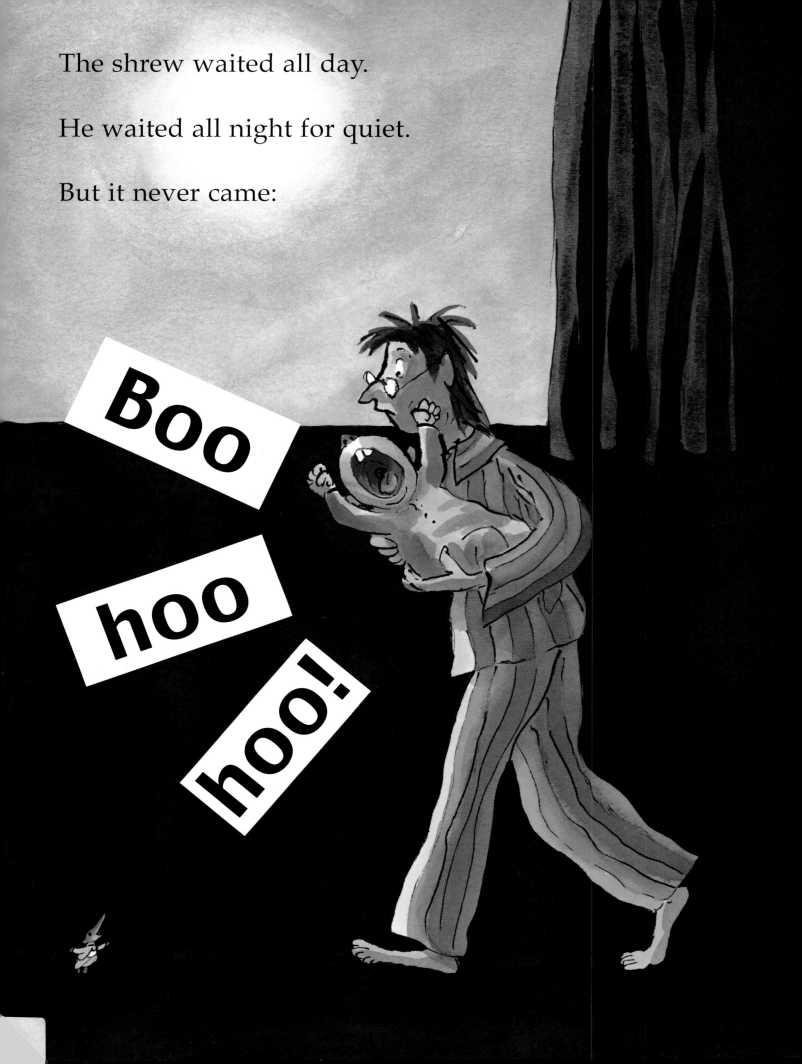

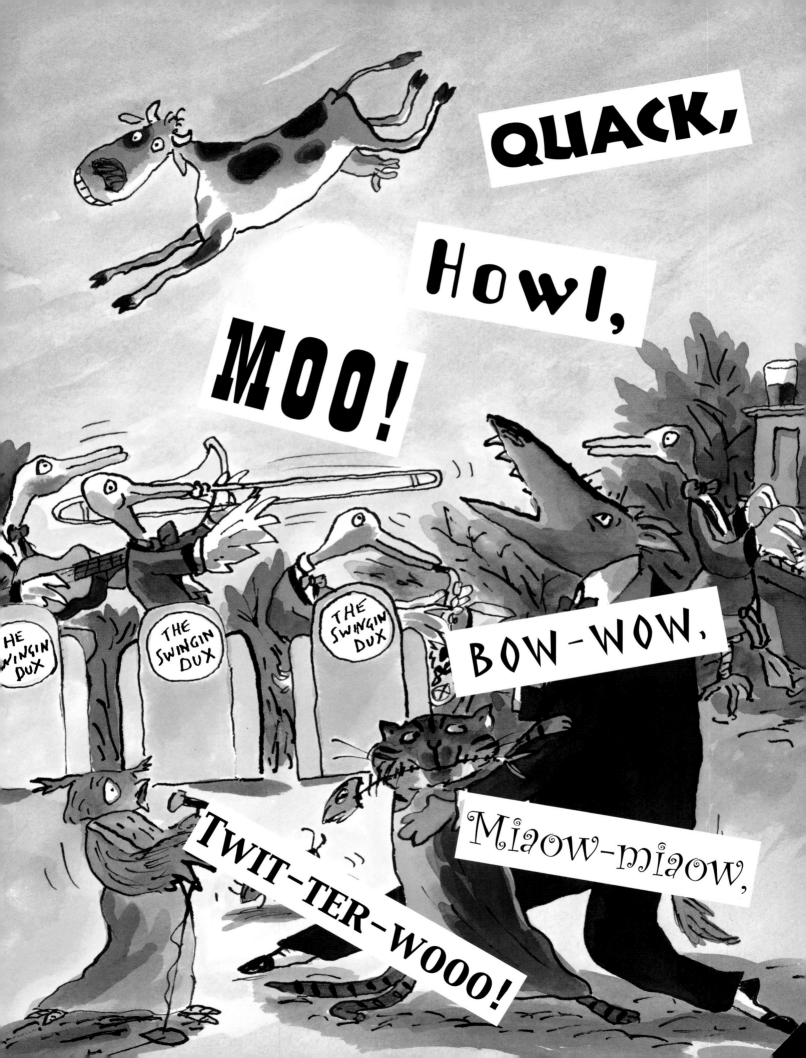

Morning came.

The shrew shouted his news from the roof.

But nobody heard him:

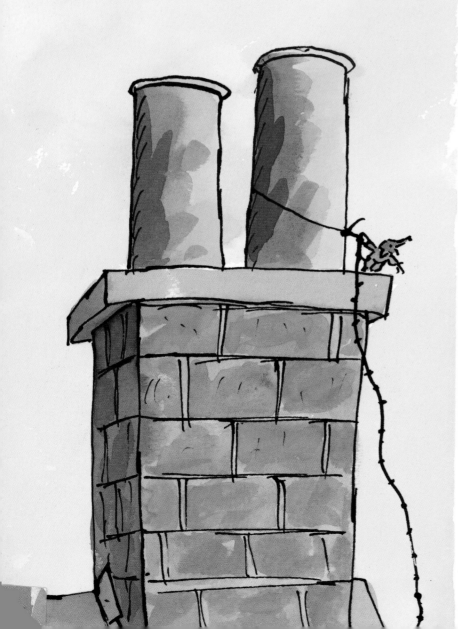
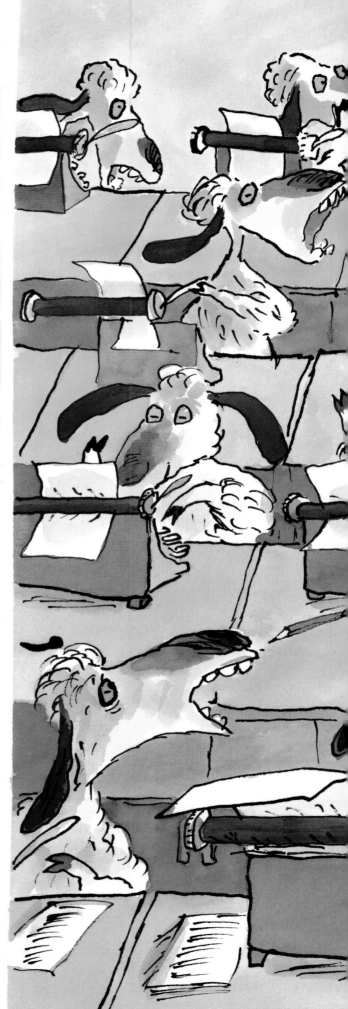

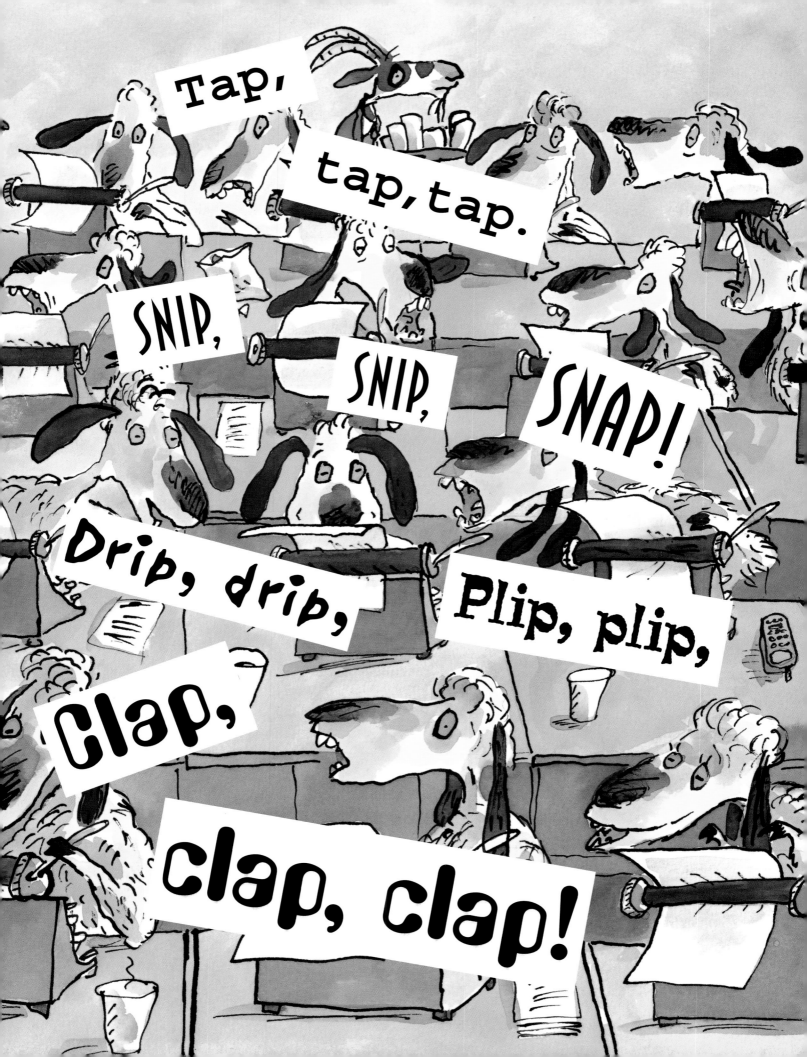

He went to the bottom of
the valley.

And tried again.

But still no one heard a word
he said:

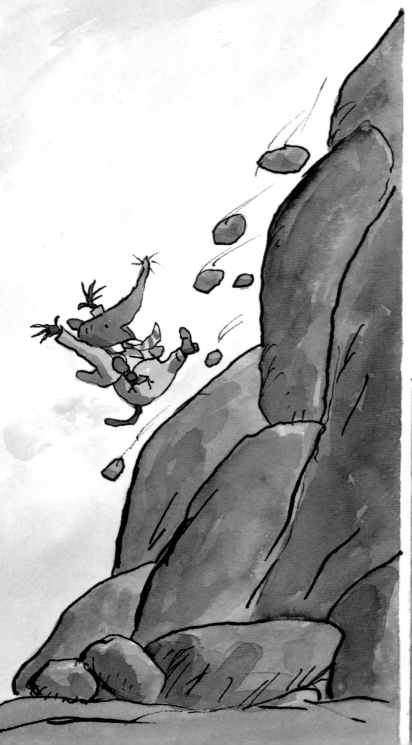
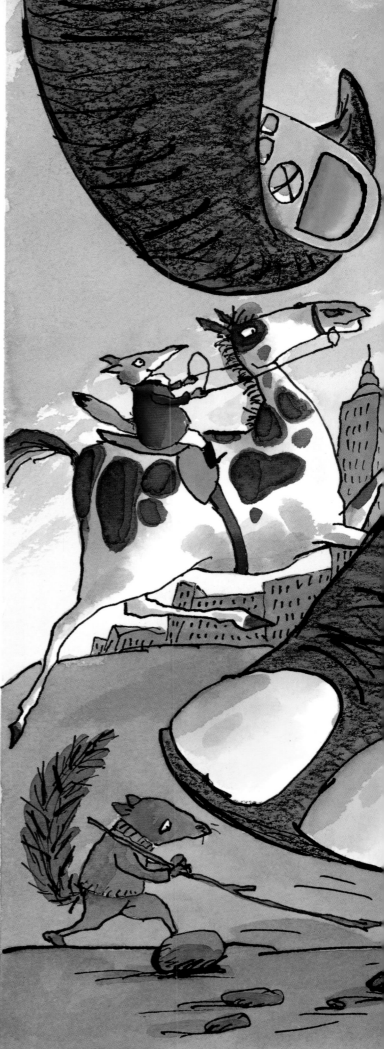

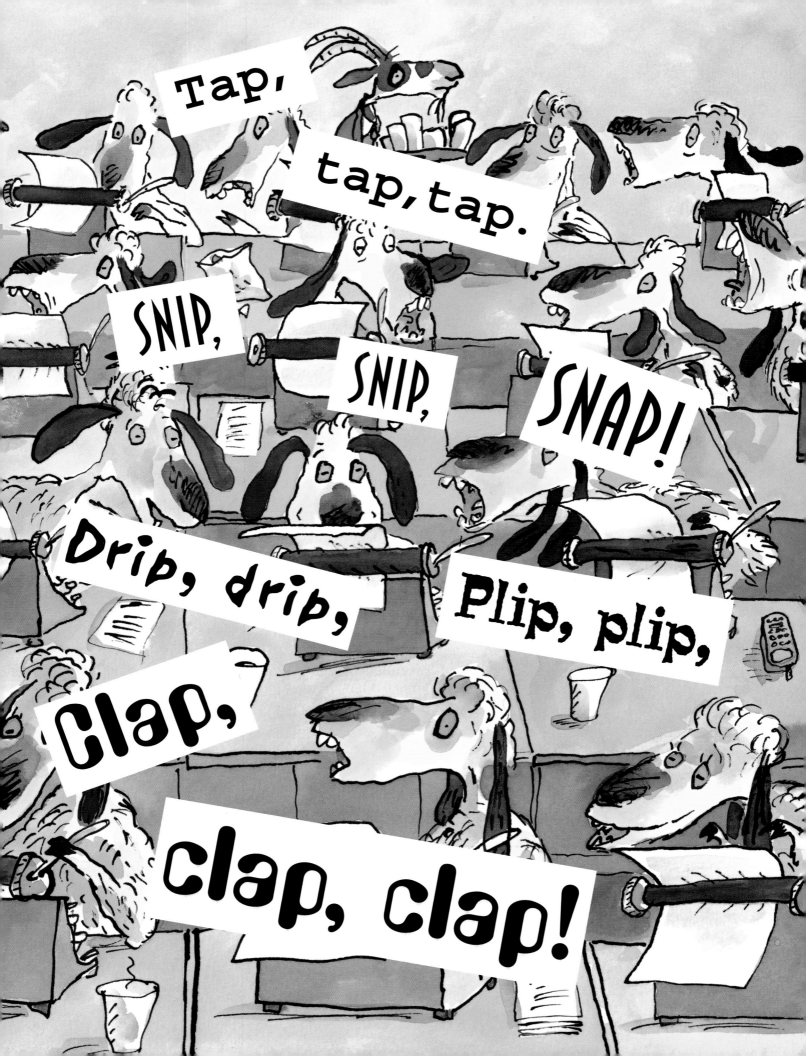

He went to the bottom of
the valley.

And tried again.

But still no one heard a word
he said:

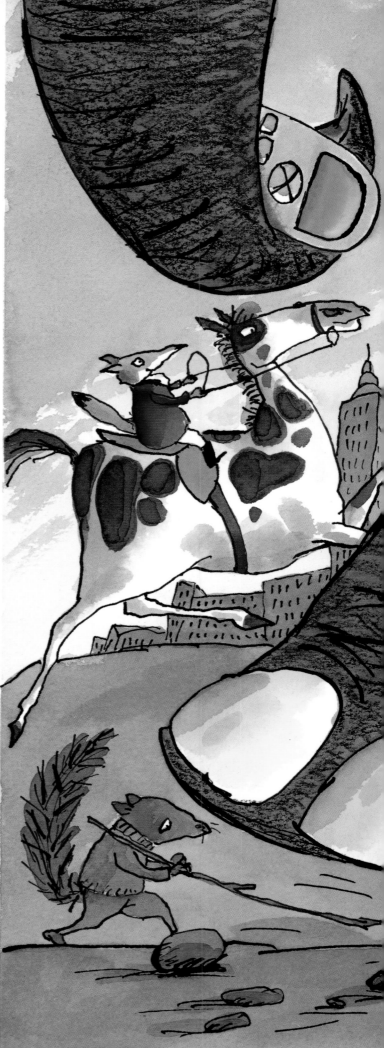
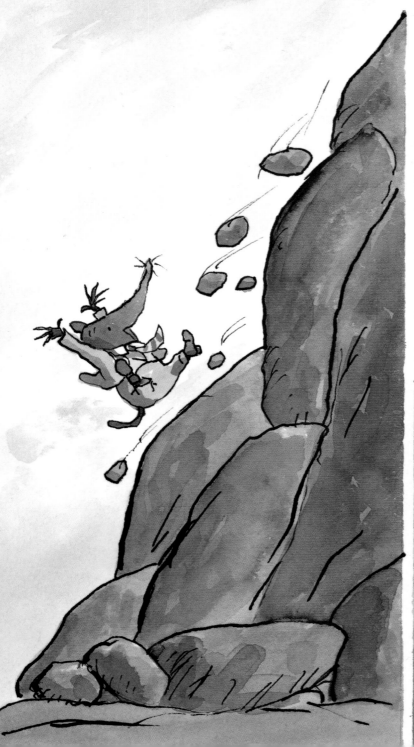

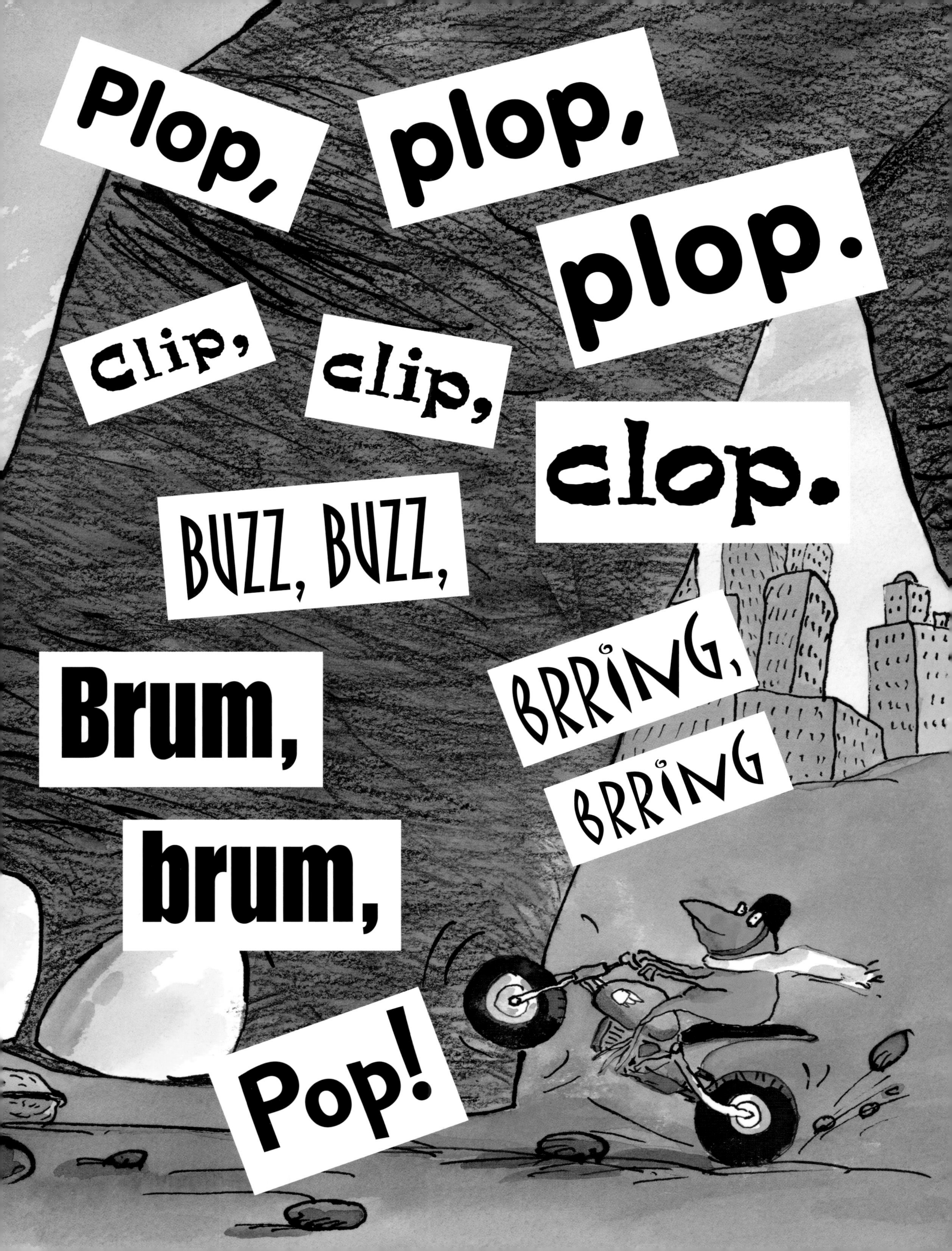
Plop, plop, plop.
clip, clip, clop.
BUZZ, BUZZ,
BRRING, BRRING
Brum, brum,
Pop!

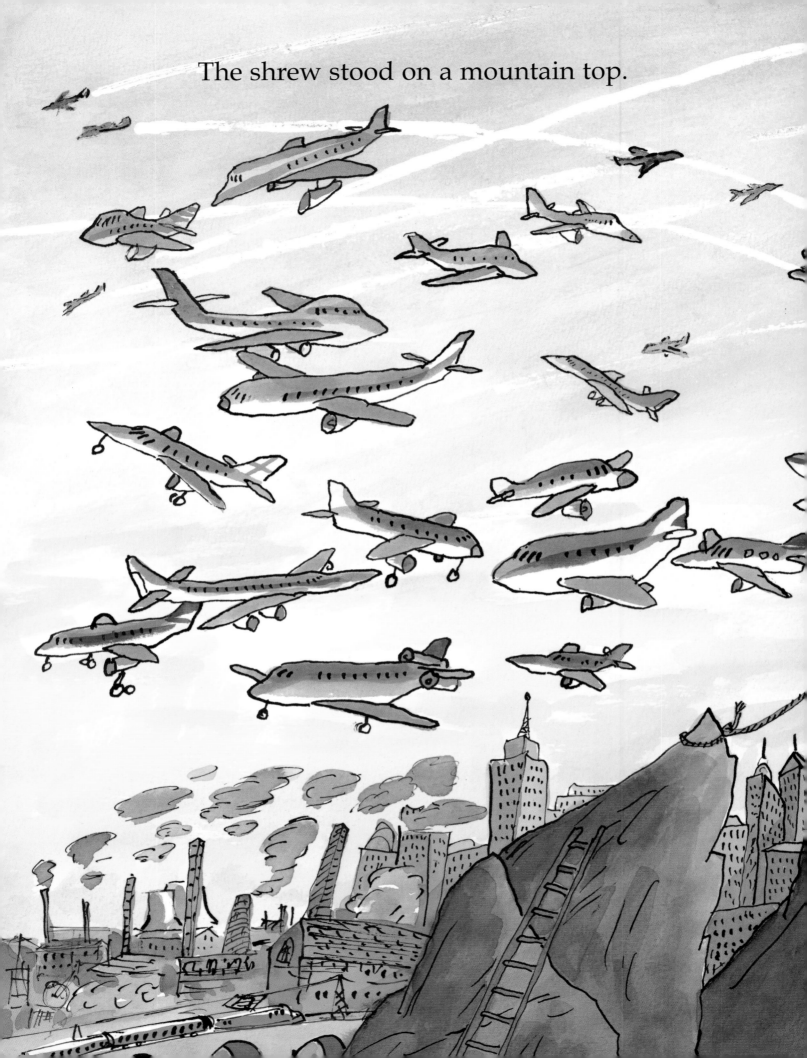

The shrew stood on a mountain top.

He threw back his
head and said,

"Shhhhhhh!
I know the secret of Peace on Earth!"

But nobody heard the shrew.
The world was too noisy:

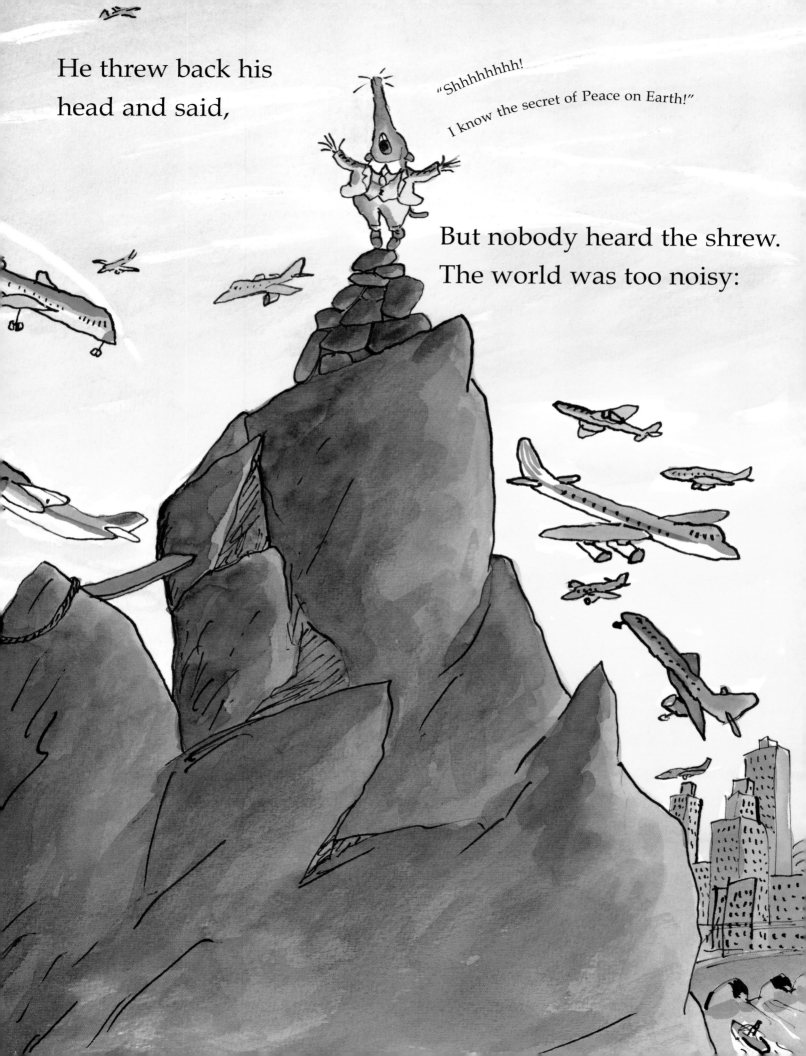

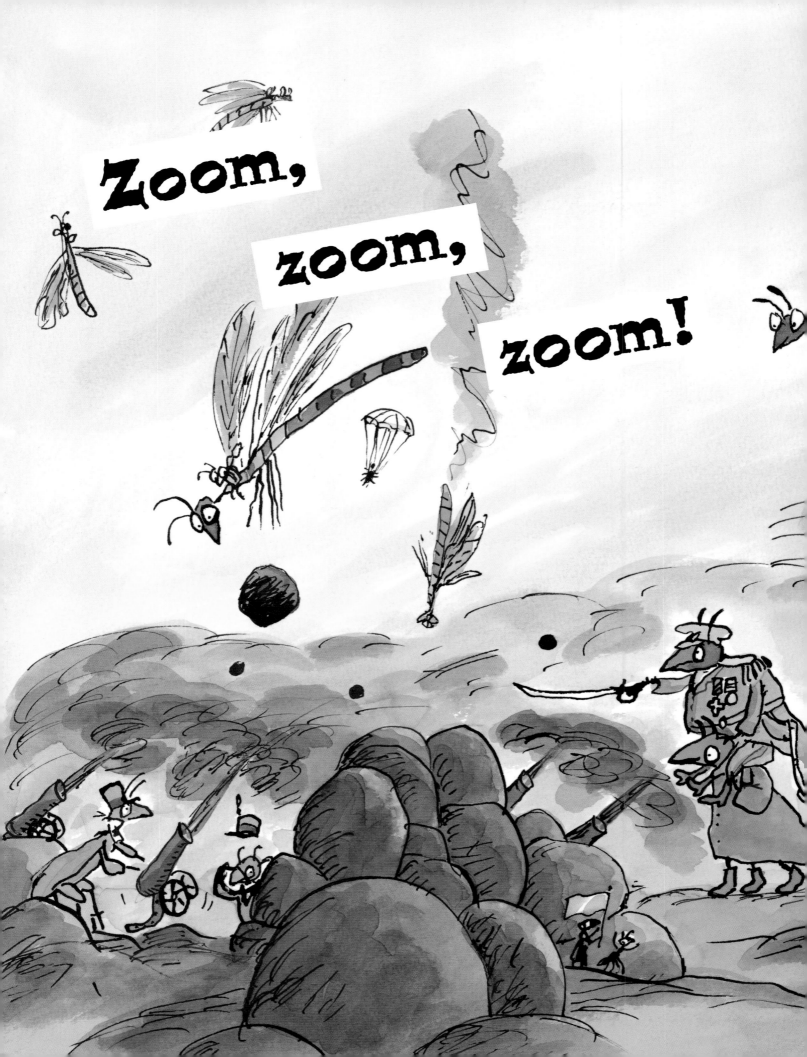

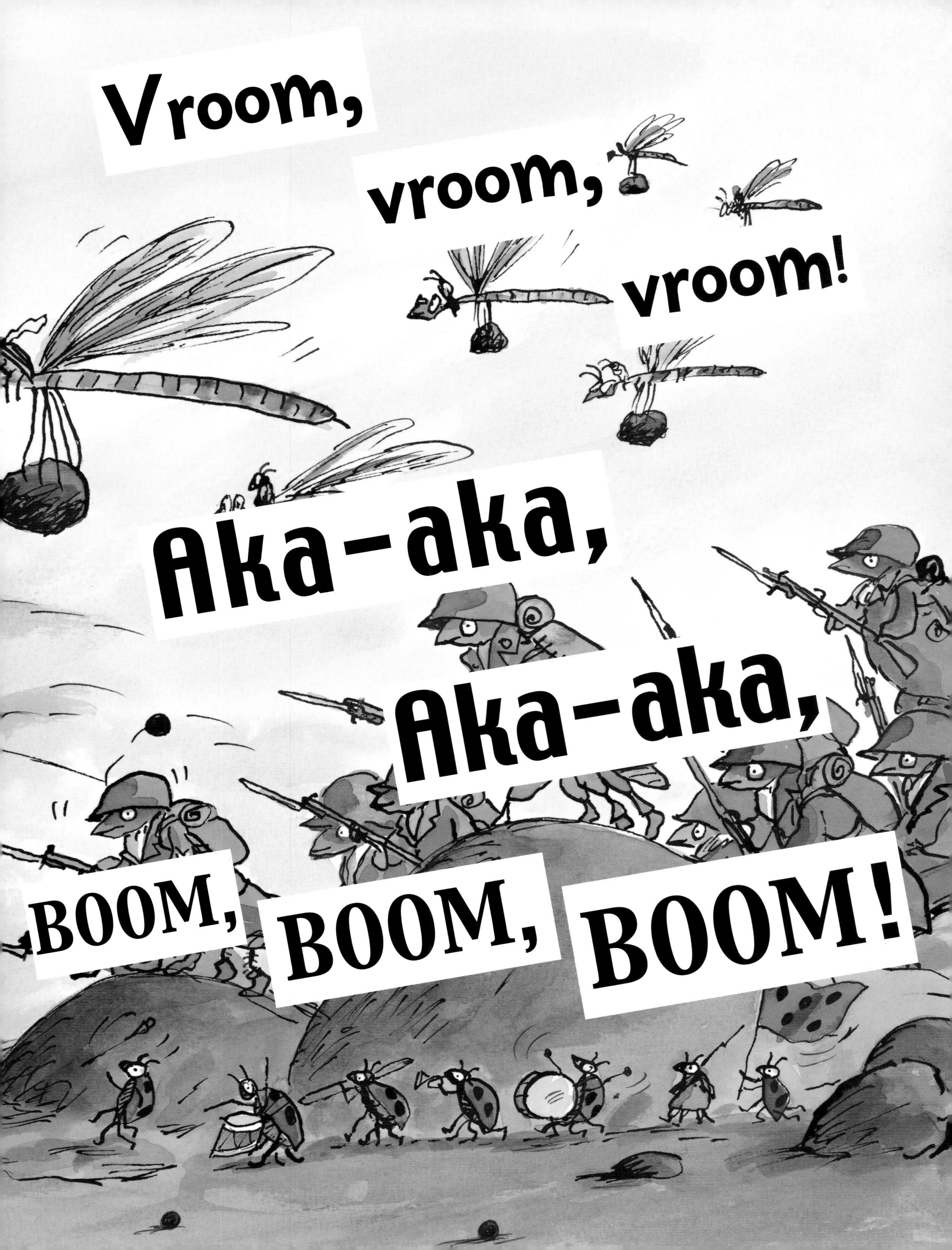
Vroom,
vroom,
vroom!
Aka-aka,
Aka-aka,
BOOM,
BOOM,
BOOM!

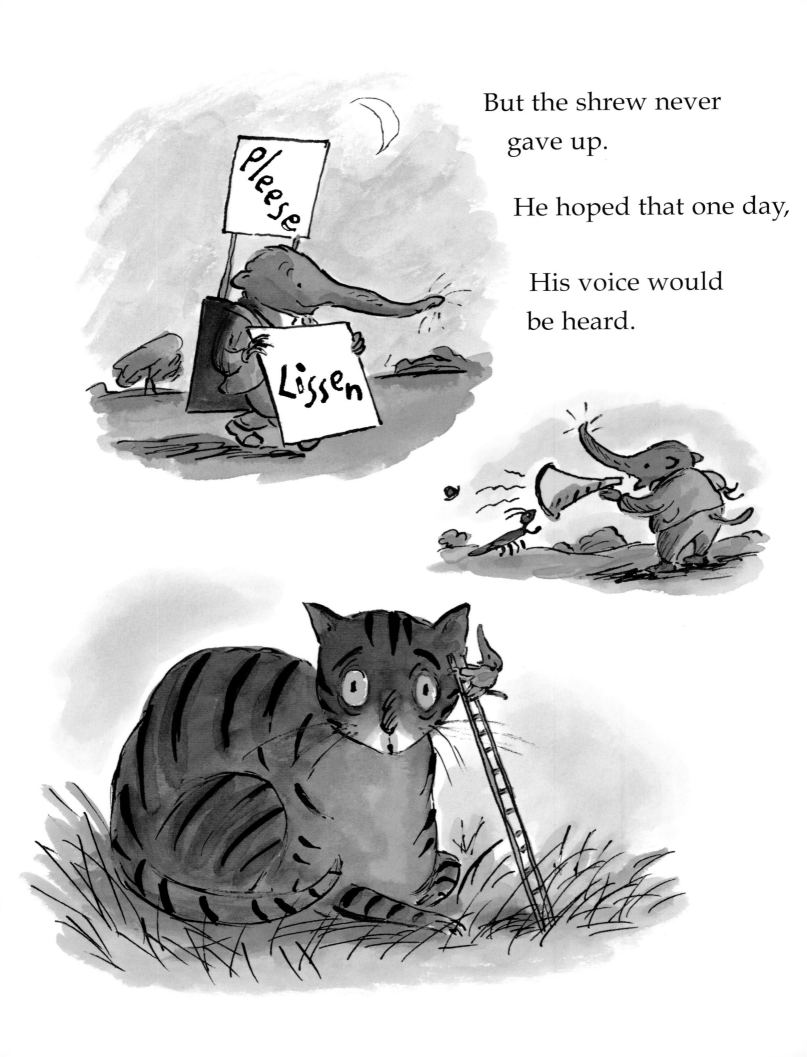

But the shrew never
gave up.

He hoped that one day,

His voice would
be heard.

Maybe if we count to three,
And keep very, very quiet,
Perhaps we will hear him.
Shall we try? Altogether now:

One, two, three . . .

Shhhhhhhhhh!

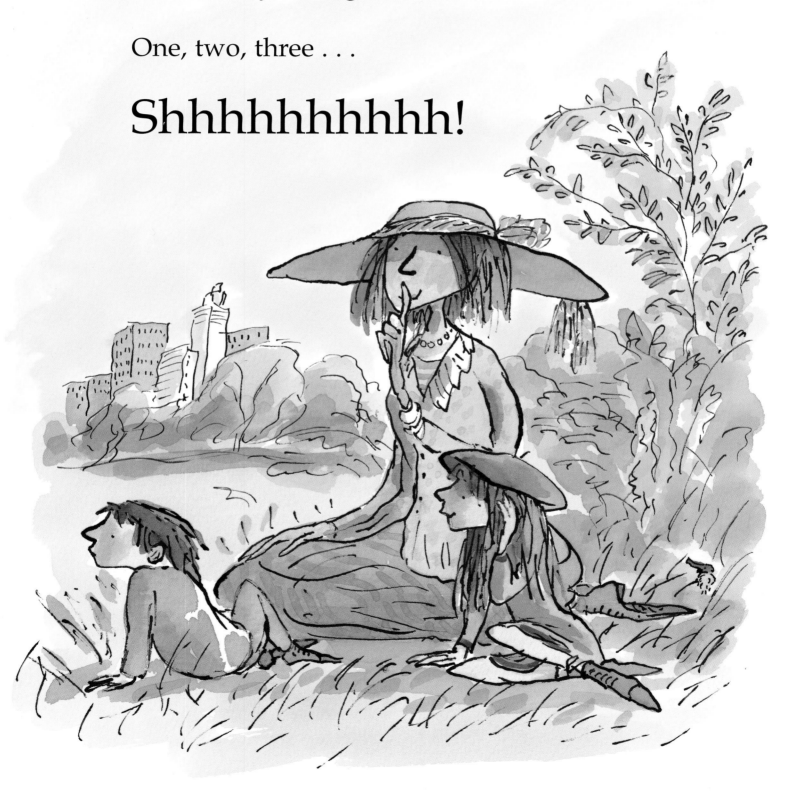

Wonderful news!
You have made a little bit of peace.

Imagine if everyone in the world
Sat still and listened just like that:

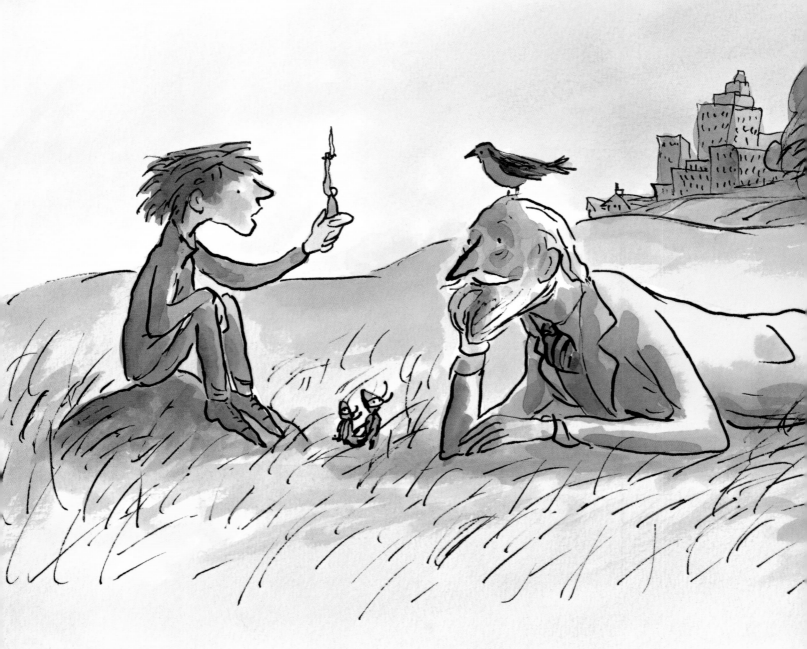

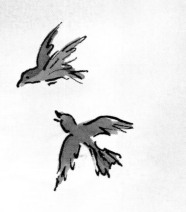

One, two, three,
Shhhhhh!

There would be Peace on Earth . . .

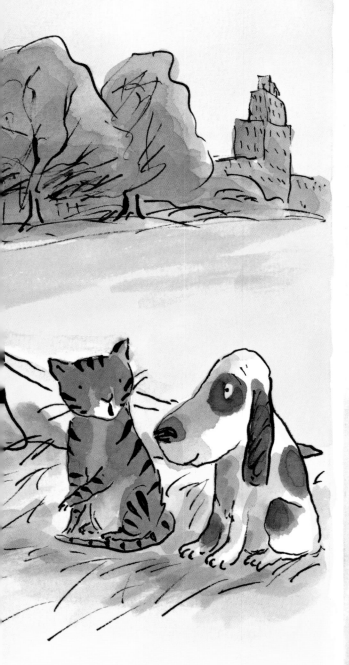

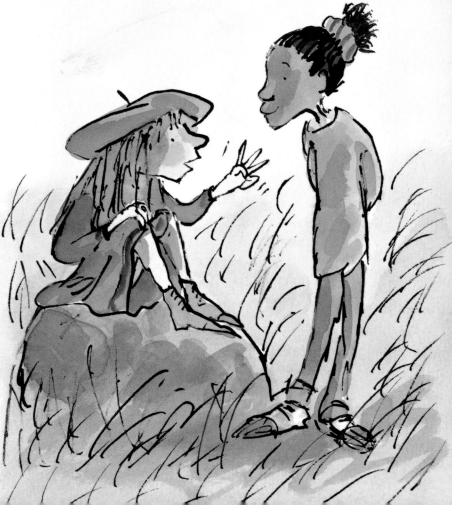

That is the secret.

Or so I've heard.

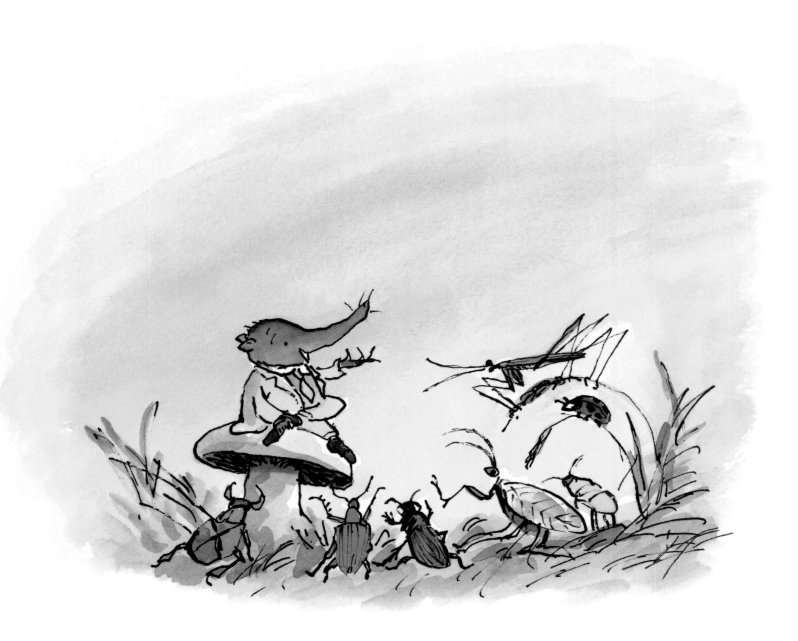

Other titles written by Jeanne Willis and illustrated by Tony Ross:

Daft Bat

Dozy Mare

I Hate School

Killer Gorilla

Manky Monkey

Misery Moo

The Really Rude Rhino

Tadpole's Promise

What Did I Look Like When I Was A Baby?

Dr Xargle's Book of Earthlets

'One of the classic picture book partnerships' Achuka